Intervention in Child Language Disorders

A Comprehensive Handbook

Ronald B. Hoodin, PhD, CCC-SLP
Speech-Language Pathology Program
Eastern Michigan University
Ypsilanti, Michigan

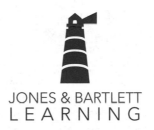

JONES & BARTLETT
L E A R N I N G

World Headquarters

Jones & Bartlett Learning	Jones & Bartlett Learning	Jones & Bartlett Learning
40 Tall Pine Drive	Canada	International
Sudbury, MA 01776	6339 Ormindale Way	Barb House, Barb Mews
978-443-5000	Mississauga, Ontario L5V 1J2	London W6 7PA
info@jblearning.com	Canada	United Kingdom
www.jblearning.com		

Jones & Bartlett Learning books and products are available through most bookstores and online book-sellers. To contact Jones & Bartlett Learning directly, call 800-832-0034, fax 978-443-8000, or visit our website, www.jblearning.com.

Production Credits
Publisher: David Cella
Associate Editor: Maro Gartside
Production Director: Amy Rose
Senior Production Editor: Renée Sekerak
Associate Production Editor: Julia Waugaman
Marketing Manager: Grace Richards
Manufacturing and Inventory Control Supervisor: Amy Bacus
Composition: Glyph International
Cover Design: Scott Moden
Cover Image: © Marilyn Volan/ShutterStock, Inc.
Printing and Binding: Malloy Incorporated
Cover Printing: Malloy Incorporated

Library of Congress Cataloging-in-Publication Data
Intervention in child language disorders :
a comprehensive handbook / edited by Ronald B. Hoodin.
   p. ; cm.
Includes bibliographical references and index.
ISBN-13: 978-0-7637-7943-6
ISBN-10: 0-7637-7943-1
1. Language disorders in children—Handbooks, manuals, etc. I. Hoodin, Ronald B.
[DNLM: 1. Language Disorders—diagnosis—Handbooks. 2. Language Disorders—therapy—Handbooks. 3. Child. 4. Language Therapy—methods—Handbooks. WL 39 I615 2011]
RJ496.L35I68 2011
618.92'855—dc22
                                2010009696
6048
Printed in the United States of America
14 13 12 11 10   10 9 8 7 6 5 4 3 2 1

Contents

Preface

This comprehensive handbook has been written for those providing treatment to children who have language disorders. It emphasizes the provision of intervention and is suitable for both practicing and student speech-language pathologists. The handbook has been divided into two portions: theoretical foundations and practical applications. Each has been subdivided into several chapters.

Even though this handbook addresses a wide range of topics in childhood language disorders, it is different from a textbook. A textbook provides a broad framework, or standard, representing a field. Each chapter presents a topic that is important in its own right. Accordingly, chapters are often lengthy, reflecting the information explosion seen in many fields, including communication disorders. By contrast, in this handbook, the purpose of which is less ambitious, topics are selected and organized on the basis that they inform or give character to the treatment activities. The information in each chapter in the theoretical foundations portion contributes to the readers' understanding of and ability to provide intervention services in the context of multiculturalism to children with language disorders. As such, this handbook has been designed to be both more focused and more readable than a textbook.

Although other treatment handbooks have been written over the years, this one is special because it is comprehensive. This handbook not only addresses a wide range of topics covered in other texts, but it also has been designed to be comprehensive with respect to several other important variables including the age of the children, the cause of the language disorder, the nature of the linguistic deficiency, and the approaches to intervention. However, there is an orientation in favor of treatments that have strong empirical support.

The practical applications portion of this handbook focuses on actual treatment for language disorders in children. The topics include planning intervention by setting goals and objectives, baselining target behaviors, selecting intervention procedures, executing the program of intervention, and evaluating the efficacy of intervention.

A second reason this handbook is unique is because treatment approaches are discussed on a conceptual level (Chapter 6) and specific treatment procedures are presented (Chapter 10). A rich array of exemplars demonstrates intervention procedures across ages, etiologies, and linguistic impairments with respect to skill acquisition and generalization. Each exemplar is generically described to improve readability and clarity. Moreover, the exemplars are individually written by experienced professionals who draw from a rich history of providing language intervention services to children. Many years of combined experience are reflected in the array of exemplars, which provide the kind of richness that comes from professional maturity. Tables included in Chapter 10 readily identify relevant exemplars. For example, a professional who is planning intervention with an infant could use the tables to identify all other exemplars with infants. An individual planning intervention that targets grammatical morphemes could use the tables to identify all exemplars that teach grammatical morphemes. Therefore, the tables serve as valuable tools for the clinician planning intervention because they classify exemplars based on salient features.

A third reason that this handbook is unique is that it has been designed in all of its dimensions to be reader friendly. The chapters are sequenced logically. Chapter Objectives are listed at the beginning and a brief Summary appears at the end of each chapter. A Glossary of terms is available. Reading the handbook cover to cover is not actually necessary. The knowledgeable reader can go straight to the topic of interest. When important terms are introduced in the text, they are bolded to highlight them. A list of terms is presented at the end of each chapter. The handbook is self-contained. Therefore, the reader will not have the chore of finding remote references to understand the text. The exemplars have been written in a consistent format to reduce the burden on the reader. Tables 10–1 and 10–2 have been constructed with the busy professional in mind. They are straightforward and readily bring the reader to relevant exemplars.

In summary, this book has been written to help children with language disorders by making clinicians more effective providers of speech-language pathology intervention.

Acknowledgments

I would like to acknowledge several sources of support in writing this book: first, my students, who energized me in the classroom with their enthusiasm for the material; second, my colleagues, who engaged me with some spirited debates in the faculty lunchroom on the professional issues; and last but perhaps most importantly, my friend and wife, Flora, who believed in me all along.

Contributors

Bill Cupples, PhD, CCC-SLP
Professor of Special Education
Eastern Michigan University

Brenda Doster, PhD, CED
Assistant Professor
Eastern Michigan University

Ana Claudia Harten, PhD, CCC-SLP
Assistant Professor
Eastern Michigan University

Denise Kowalski, MA, CCC-SLP
Clinical Educator
Eastern Michigan University

Linda J. Polter, MA, SpA, CED
Associate Professor
Eastern Michigan University

Lizbeth Curme Stevens, PhD, CCC-SLP
Associate Professor
Eastern Michigan University

Reviewers

Jennifer C. Friberg, EdD, CCC-SLP/SRCL
Assistant Professor
Illinois State University

Monica Gordon Pershey, EdD, CCC-SLP
Associate Professor, Program Director
Department of Health Sciences
Cleveland State University

Patricia Hargrove, PhD
Professor
Minnesota State University, Mankato

Anthony Pak Hin Kong, PhD
Assistant Professor
Department of Communication Sciences and Disorders
University of Central Florida

Adrienne McElroy-Bratcher, SLPD, CCC-SLP
Assistant Professor
Department of Communicative Disorders
Eastern New Mexico University

Debra Schober-Peterson, PhD, CCC-SLP
Clinical Associate Professor
Georgia State University

Suzanne H. Swift, EdD, CCC-SLP
Chair, Department of Health and Human Services
Associate Professor of Communication Disorders
Eastern New Mexico University

CHAPTER 1

Introduction

Ronald B. Hoodin

Chapter Objectives

After reading this chapter, you should be able to:

- Discuss the difference between communication and language.
- Discuss the difference between symbolic and nonsymbolic communication.
- Discuss the notion of communicative intent.
- Define the concept of language.
- Identify and describe the receptive and expressive language modalities.
- Identify and describe the linguistic parameters.

Most children grow up and acquire speech and language without requiring individualized, professional help. However, some children, for a variety of reasons, do not achieve communicative proficiency on their own. Consequently, their ability to get their needs met by interacting with others and engaging in activities is undermined. Moreover, these children often become socially isolated with severe consequences. This book is written on behalf of these children and for the professionals charged with helping them.

In this first chapter, the foundation is provided for the remainder of the book. The basic concepts of communication, speech, and language are introduced and elaborated on. Providing this background for the reader serves as a foundation for understanding the later topics, including language acquisition, language disorders, and, of course, language intervention, the most important topic in this book.

Communication

Communication is pervasive in life. Birds sing. Lions roar. Dogs bark. Human infants cry. Each sends a message. **Communication** refers to the exchange of information (McLaughlin, 1998). There is a sender, a receiver, and the information exchanged. Although other creatures communicate, the focus of this book is on human communication. Human communication has been traced back to the mists of time.

Symbolic and Nonsymbolic Communication

Human communication need not be symbolic. To communicate symbolically, the speaker uses a **symbol** to stand for something else, its referent. The relationship between the symbol and the referent is arbitrary. That is, the symbol does not resemble the referent. Rather, the two are tied by community consensus. For example, the word *lion* is a symbol for a large, ferocious feline. However, there is no resemblance between the word *lion* and that large, ferocious feline. A lion is called a lion simply because those in the linguistic community call it a lion. An example of nonsymbolic human communication would be when a hungry 2-day-old infant cries and the mother responds by making an accurate assessment of why her baby is distressed and provides nourishment. Clearly, the child has communicated. The sender (infant) transmitted the information to the receiver (mother). However, the crying directly communicated the distress of hunger. At this young age, the infant did not use crying to symbolize hunger. Instead, crying was an aspect of the distress the hungry child was experiencing.

Communicative Intent

During the first year of life, a child typically develops **communicative intent** (Hulit & Howard, 2006). The child demonstrates that he or she means to communicate by his or her behavior. A child may point toward a cookie while vocalizing and gazing back and forth between the caretaker's face and the cookie. If the caretaker does not respond immediately to the request for the cookie, then the child will likely persist. By persisting, the sender expects the receiver to take note. The child possesses communicative intent. Interestingly, people report similar behaviors in their dogs and cats, which suggest that these animals also have communicative intent. For example, when someone approaches a dog's food, the dog may growl menacingly while glaring at the person and baring its teeth. This behavior may persist, signaling the unambiguous warning, "stay away or else."

Had the child in the cookie example been about 2 years old, he or she may have said, "eat cookie" to request the cookie. In making the request using words, the child has actually used language. The child has uttered a primitive sentence. The sentence is devoid of grammatical markers and includes only substantive words. Nonetheless, it is a linguistic message. As shown, a child may communicate the message either linguistically (eat + cookie) or nonlinguistically (vocalize + point + gaze coupling). Both forms of human communication are common.

Language

Now that communication has been defined, the concept of language will be addressed. From a linguistic perspective, **language** refers to a system of symbols and rules for combining these symbols to communicate a message (Hegde, 2001). Language has a generative quality, which means that with a finite set of symbols and a finite set of rules for combining these symbols, an individual may express an infinite number of correct utterances. That is, the symbols are combined and recombined in numerous ways to send messages. Therefore, when a child says a primitive utterance, such as "eat cookie," he or she may not be simply parroting an adult but instead may be engaged in the creative act of uttering a sentence that never existed before, at least for this child.

Linguistic Modalities

Symbolic communication, or language, facilitates human communication. The entire world (objects, events, emotions, etc.) is **mapped** linguistically by labeling (symbolizing) each concept with a word. Then, theoretically at least, individuals put their thoughts into linguistic form and send any imaginable message to others. The process of putting messages into linguistic form is referred to as **formulating language**, or encoding. The language to be conveyed is called **expressive language**. Once the message has been formulated linguistically, individuals can convey the message to others. One option, or expressive modality, is to use speech. **Speaking** refers to using the **vocal tract**, or speech structures, to express the linguistic message. Other expressive modalities include writing and gesturing, as in American Sign Language.

Another person receives the message using the receptive modalities. The receptive modalities include listening to spoken language, reading written language, and feeling gestural language by touch. Feeling gestural language by touch is not often mentioned; however, it represents a viable receptive modality for the deaf–blind population. Braille is also received through touch. The message receiver is said to decode, or **interpret**, the linguistic message. As such, the sender formulates, or encodes, the message, whereas the receiver interprets, or decodes, the message. The language the receiver interprets is called **receptive language**. When individuals are impaired in receptive or expressive language, they are at a distinct disadvantage in life. However, by strategizing, it is sometimes possible to compensate by relying more heavily on an intact modality to reduce dependence on an impaired modality. For example, hearing-impaired children may acquire speech-reading skills to augment visually their residual hearing abilities. This compensatory strategy may improve their success in communicating.

Speech and Language as Communicative Tools

The role of speech and language has been placed in the broader perspective of communication by a model called the speech chain (Denes & Pinson, 1993). According to this model, the message starts off as an idea in the mind of the speaker (cognitive realm) and undergoes numerous transformations: encoded into language (linguistic realm), sent along the nervous system to move the speech structures (physiologic realm), transmitted through the airways as sound waves (acoustic realm), impacted on the listener's ear to stimulate the ascending auditory pathways (physiologic realm), organized at the cerebral cortex into language (linguistic realm), and, finally, decoded into a message (cognitive realm) in the mind of the listener. The message then has gone full circle. What started as an idea in the mind of the speaker went through numerous transformations and ended up as an idea in the mind of the listener. It is apparent from this model that all of the information in the speaker's message has to be represented in each transformation, including in speech and language. Speech and language serve in this model as communicative tools. Furthermore, when a child requests a cookie from an adult and gets it, the child's use of communication as a behavior has been strengthened. The converse is also true. When a child requests a cookie and the request is ignored, communication as a behavior has been weakened.

Linguistic Parameters

For professionals interested in fostering language development in children, simply knowing the definitions of language and related terminology is insufficient. Consequently, they have turned to the linguistic parameters to gain further insight into a child's language proficiency. Linguists have identified different parameters that occur simultaneously during speech (McLaughlin, 1998). Language consists of five parameters: (1) phonology, (2) semantics, (3) syntax, (4) morphology, and (5) pragmatics, which are defined next. Children can fall behind their peers in any one or more of the **linguistic parameters**. Therefore, each parameter represents a vehicle for viewing the child's language level and for monitoring language development.

Phonology refers to the sounds of spoken language. It includes the individual speech sounds or the consonants and vowels that differentiate words and are called **phonemes**. Phonology also includes the **prosodic features**, stress, intonation, and rhythm. The prosodic features are sound patterns that can only be identified when listening to the overall utterance, and they cannot be perceived by listening to individual phonemes. **Stress** is the extra strength or loudness placed on some linguistic unit like a syllable or word. **Intonation** is the pitch envelope over the utterance, and **rhythm** refers to the stress timing, or the beat, of spoken language.

The parameter called **semantics** addresses the meaning of language. It includes word meaning and much more. For example, everyone understands the meaning of the sentence, "The grass is green." But the following makes no sense "grass the green is," even though the same words are used. Consequently, it is apparent that in a sentence there is meaning that exceeds the mere meaning of individual words. This basic or underlying meaning arising out of the sentence is called *propositional meaning*.

Syntax refers to the rules of word order. Syntactic rules apply on the sentence, clause, and phrase levels. An example of a syntactic rule follows: A kernel sentence has the basic subject + verb + object order (e.g., *The dog chased the ball*). However, by changing word order (exchanging places between the subject and object noun and making other changes), this kernel sentence has been transformed into the passive sentence, "The ball was chased by the dog." The passive form emphasizes what was done rather than who did it.

Morphology is the parameter that concerns the rules for using word forms and inflections. A **morpheme** is the smallest linguistic unit to have meaning. There are two types of morphemes: lexical and bound morphemes. In the phrase "The baby's rattle," there are four morphemes and they have been underlined. Three of the morphemes (*the, baby, rattle*) are called lexical morphemes because they are part of the lexicon, or vocabulary. The possessive marker *s* is called a **bound morpheme** because it has to be bound, or attached, to a lexical morpheme to have meaning.

Pragmatics concerns the rules that govern language in a social context. Its reach is broad and inclusive and ranges from such diverse topics as using politeness markers (*please, thank you*, etc.), to taking turns in conversations, and to repairing conversations that have broken down.

As children develop and become more mature, they are expected to become more proficient linguistically. Linguistic development occurs in each of the parameters of language. As time passes, most children speak more clearly, use more complex grammatical forms, send more nuanced messages, and engage more skillfully in conversations. However, some children fall behind their peers in one or more of the linguistic parameters, with unfortunate consequences. These children need to be identified and helped so they can lead more productive, less isolated lives. Helping these children develop linguistically is the topic of this handbook.

Most children acquire language relatively autonomously through exposure. However, a caring and knowledgeable adult can facilitate language development. Because of the serious negative consequences of not developing linguistic proficiency, speech-language pathologists and others have tried to develop intervention approaches to help these children. Such thinking has led clinicians to reflect consciously on the nature of language. This ability to reflect on language is called **metalinguistics**. Fostering the development of metalinguistic skills in children may actually enhance their language development. However, sufficient cognitive development is a prerequisite to the acquisition of metalinguistic skills.

Chapter Summary

The concepts of speech and language are discussed and placed in the broader communication perspective. The expressive and receptive language modalities are described, and the linguistic parameters are identified. These basic concepts are related to language acquisition and language disorders. Although most children acquire language without individual professional help, other children do not progress sufficiently to keep up with their typically developing peers. Children who need extra help acquiring language represent the focus of this book.

Terms from the Chapter

Bound morpheme *(5)*
Communication *(2)*
Communicative intent *(2)*
Expressive language *(3)*
Formulating language *(3)*
Interpreting language *(4)*
Intonation *(5)*
Language *(3)*
Linguistic parameters *(5)*
Mapping *(3)*
Metalinguistics *(6)*
Morpheme *(5)*
Morphology *(5)*

Phoneme *(5)*
Phonology *(5)*
Pragmatics *(6)*
Prosodic features *(5)*
Receptive language *(4)*
Rhythm *(5)*
Semantics *(5)*
Speaking *(3)*
Stress *(5)*
Symbol *(2)*
Syntax *(5)*
Vocal tract *(3)*

INTRODUCTION

References

Denes, P. B., & Pinson, E. N. (1993). *The speech chain: The physics and biology of spoken language*. New York, NY: W. H. Freeman.

Hegde, M. N. (2001). *Introduction to communication disorders* (3rd ed.). Austin, TX: PRO-Ed.

Hulit, L. M., & Howard, M. R. (2006). *Born to talk: An introduction to speech and language development* (4th ed.). Boston, MA: Pearson.

McLaughlin, S. (1998). *Introduction to language development*. San Diego, CA: Singular Publishing Group.

C H A P T E R 2

Overview of Language Acquisition

Lizbeth Curme Stevens

Chapter Objectives

After reading this chapter, you should be able to:

- Identify and explain factors in language development.
- Describe milestones of language development in the infant (birth through 2 years).
- Describe milestones of language development in the preschool-age child from 3 through 5 years.
- Describe milestones of language development in school-age children.
- Discuss milestones in acquisition of written language (reading, writing, and spelling).
- Discuss implications of language development for intervention.

In the introductory chapter, you were provided with a framework for the process of communication (Denes & Pinson, 1993). As indicated, language is but one component of human communication (Hegde, 2001). Its development seems to occur effortlessly in most children. When delays occur, the whole communication system is potentially at risk. Understanding key factors and milestones in the development of communication and specifically in the acquisition of language should guide us in our efforts to address language disorders.

The purpose of this chapter is to survey factors contributing to language development, as well as general characteristics and major milestones of language acquisition across the child's age span. This chapter is not intended to teach the readers language acquisition; rather, it is designed to provide a context for later topics, including

9

language disorders, language assessment, and language intervention. In the interest of brevity, descriptions of specific theories of language acquisition will be omitted. An overview of acquisition of linguistic form, content, and use will be included with specific examples of each. Charts of major milestones in language development will include detailed examples in all categories. For additional information, the reader is encouraged to review one of the numerous comprehensive texts devoted exclusively to language acquisition. The intent of this chapter is to frame our role as agents of prevention and intervention through our discussion and understanding of normal language acquisition processes. Knowledge of contributing factors to the orderly development of language may permit us to assist in supporting the language learning process when for some reason the system is not working.

Language Development Overview

The development of language is presumed to be innate and involves the interplay between nature and nurture. Researchers in many scientific disciplines, including education, developmental psychology, linguistics, linguistic anthropology, neuroscience, psycholinguistics, and speech-language pathology, have posed questions concerning how language is learned. Numerous theories have attempted to explain the process; however, disagreement remains about the precise nature of language learning. Currently, experts in child language are broadly divided into two groups: those who believe language learning is primarily due to genetic mechanisms activated by language input (i.e., the innate account; Pinker, 1984) and those who believe that language learning is not innate but results from actual cognitive processing of this linguistic input (i.e., the connectionist or cognitive approach; Johnston, 2007). In either case, it is clear that language input is critical in acquiring language as well as cognitive and sensory processing.

In fact, there is widespread agreement that human growth and experience affect language development within the following domains: social, perceptual, cognitive processing, conceptual, and linguistic (Johnston, 2007). According to Haynes and Shulman (1994), communication development is thought to depend on a foundation of five interrelated systems, which collectively are termed the *BACIS* (pronounced as *basis*): (1) an intact *biological system* (i.e., normal speech and hearing, a normal neurological system), (2) _access_ to models of language form and use, (3) intact _cognitive_ development, (4) _intent_ to communicate, and (5) _social development_.

In conclusion, there appears then to be a biological, cognitive, and social foundation for speech, language, and communication development. Intact auditory-vocal functioning, a normally developing nervous system, and intact cognitive processing, as well as exposure to linguistic input through child–caretaker interaction provide the basis. If an infant is born with hearing loss or a genetic condition associated with intellectual disability (e.g., Down syndrome, autism spectrum disorder (ASD), and fragile X syndrome), then the development of language and speech may be affected. Certain environmental conditions (e.g., minimal nurturing or language stimulation, which orphans may experience) may likewise affect or alter typical language development. If any of these factors are absent or deficient, then typical language development may be affected. Consequently, our understanding and knowledge of the role each factor plays is important for intervention as well as prevention.

Milestones of Language Development in the Infant (Birth Through 2 Years)

Infants are born with the necessary biological functions to learn language as described previously. During their first year of life, language emerges because of exposure to language models, interaction with humans who provide support for language learning and communication, and increasing maturation of the sensory and nervous systems and corresponding cognitive development. Once the first word has appeared (typically at 1 year), children show marked progress in their communication skill and language development through age 2 years, as the form, content, and use of language expand. These accomplishments and contributing factors are briefly reviewed:

> Learning to talk is one of the most visible and important achievements of early childhood. In a matter of months, and without explicit teaching toddlers move from hesitant single words to fluent sentences, and from a small vocabulary to one that is growing by six new words a day. New language tools mean new opportunities

for social understanding; for learning about the world; and for sharing experiences, pleasures, and needs. (Johnston, 2007, p. 1)

Infants communicate through reflexive cries and other vocalizations. This behavior is termed **perlocutionary** as it is unintended, not deliberate, and does not involve symbolism. These vocalizations, however, affect the mother who interprets them and responds accordingly (Owens, 2008). The infant learns, then, over time that the mother or other caring adults in the environment respond to vocalizations, which eventually results in the infant's purposeful use of them. These vocalizations and other behavior become **illocutionary** because they are intended and symbolic yet not linguistic. Joint (i.e., shared) reference, which is developing at this time, is instrumental to the communication process and later to the emergence of language. In joint or shared reference, the infant and caregiver may differentiate some action, object, or event to communicate about in various ways, including eye gaze, vocalization, pointing, or gesture. Finally, with the expression of words, the child's communication behavior becomes **locutionary**. The child now conveys messages purposefully with language forms. The role of the infant's caregivers is instrumental in this evolution through their responsiveness and assignment of meaning to the infant's behavior, even where none exists. It is through engaging in daily routines, primarily with the mother, that language eventually emerges.

At the same time, the infant's ability to explore the environment increases, which contributes to ongoing cognitive development. The stage of cognitive development ascribed to the infant between 0 and 2 years is termed *sensorimotor*, during which the concepts of causality and object permanence emerge (Piaget, 1954). During this stage, the child learns by manipulating objects and various other activities, which results in both comprehension and expression of new words facilitated by **joint reference**. In summary, the child's exposure to the environment, in concert with his or her interaction with adults, contributes to the emergence and growth of language. It is beyond the scope of this chapter to detail all aspects of cognitive development Jean Piaget postulated. The interested reader is encouraged to review other sources for more detail.

Speech appears during the first year of life, with final refinement of sound production occurring during the early school-age years. First vocalizations are reflexive and not specifically tied to language input.

See **Table 2–1** for a detailed account of phonological development and language production and comprehension during the first year of life. Broad milestones in speech development include cooing, babbling, echolalia, jargon, and phonetically consistent forms, which are wordlike approximations. The interested reader is directed to other more comprehensive texts for specific descriptions of phonological development in particular as well as other areas (lexical and pragmatic development). (See references.) It is beyond the scope of this handbook to detail the many nuances of language development in infants and young children.

The first true word emerges around 12 months. Typically, first words are nouns, across all languages, and the names of people or objects in the child's environment. These words are initially used functionally to gain attention or to make requests. The child's lexicon (i.e., his or her individually acquired "dictionary" of words and meanings) continues to expand greatly in the second year of life to add many other functions, such as describing. The number of words used expressively increases from a single word at 12 months to more than 200 words by age 2 years. A vocabulary spurt occurs in the child's second year between 18 and 24 months, most noticeably in receptive vocabulary and usually when the child has acquired 100 words (Owens, 2008). The meanings of these early words may not necessarily match adult meaning. **Overextension** refers to assigning overly broad meanings to a word; for example, calling all men "Daddy." In contrast, with **underextension**, a child may apply a restricted meaning to a word. The child may use *cup* to refer only to his or her particular cup and no others (Owens, 2008).

Similarly, as the child's vocabulary expands so does morphology and syntax. From single-word utterances at 1 year, the child moves rapidly into two- and three-word combinations. Early language development has typically been described as stages, which are defined by the average number of words, or morphemes, per utterance (i.e., the **mean length of utterance (MLU)**) and type(s) of sentence pattern used (Owens, 2008). Utterance length is determined both by the number of words and any other accompanying **grammatical morphemes** (e.g., *cuts* equals two morphemes, one for *cat* and one for plural *s*). Obligatory grammatical morphemes occurring early in language development include both affixes (e.g., past *-ed*), as well as specific words signaling advances in complexity of utterance form (e.g., introduction of auxiliary *is*). See **Table 2–2** for an overview of early development of language form. Additional highlights of form development, in addition to other

Table 2–1 Milestones of Language Development in Infants (Birth Through 1 Year)

Age	Form		Content	Use	
	Phonology		Semantics	Pragmatics	
				Perlocutionary Stage (~0–8 mos.)	
	Comprehension	Production			
Birth	Discriminate languages by rhythm	Reflexive/ vegetative sounds	Startle response, look toward sound source	Prefer infant-directed speech; start to attend to social partners	
2 Months	Distinguish own language from others	Cooing, gooing	Briefly hold, mouth, inspect objects	Aware of strangers, look at people briefly	
4 Months	Distinguish languages from same rhythmic class	Vowel sounds, squeals, growls	Distinguish purposeful from accidental actions; object category formation begins	Recognize own name; fix gaze on faces	
6 Months	Discriminate between allophones of same phoneme [disappears at 11 months]; segment words and clausal units in fluent speech	Reduplicated babbling appears (e.g., *bababa*)	Understand "no"; attempt imitation of gestures	Engage in joint attention	

Illocutionary Stage (~ 8–12 mos.)

8 Months	Discriminate between stress and phonotactic patterns of own language and others; attend to fine phonetic detail	Variegated babbling appears (e.g., *babigaba*) Child imitates adult vocalizations (9 mos.)	Look in correct place for objects out of sight and search for partially hidden ones	Onset of intentional communication; preverbal language functions appear: attention seeking, requesting, greeting, transferring, protesting or rejecting, responding or acknowledging, and informing; gestures used to communicate (8 or 9 mos.)
10–12 Months	Identify function words (e.g., *a, the*) in utterances	Use jargon in babbling; produce first word	Understand means–end; understand 5–10 words; produce first word; responds to about half of mother's verbal and nonverbal requests (11 mos.)	Use imperative pointing (10 mos.); produce first word (**marks onset of locutionary stage**)

Source: Adapted from Owens, 2008; Pence & Justice, 2008.

Table 2–2 Brown's Stages of Language Development

Stage	MLU	Age in Months (approximate)	Characteristics (Note: morpheme mastery is upper limit of age range; some children master forms earlier)
I	1.0–2.0	12–26	Linear semantic rules (single word usage)
II	2.0–2.5	27–30	Morphological development; all 14 morphemes appear; morphemes mastered: *on, in, ing*
III	2.5–3.0	31–34	Sentence-form development Morphemes mastered: plural *-s*
IV	3.0–3.75	35–40	Embedding Morphemes mastered: possessive *'s*, uncontractible copula (e.g., *He is* (in response to "who's sick?"))
V	3.75–4.5	41–46	Joining clauses (compound sentences) Morphemes mastered: irregular past, articles (*a, the*), third person singular *-s*
V+	4.5+	47+	Morphemes mastered: regular past *-ed*, irregular third person (*does, has*), uncontractible auxiliary (e.g., *He is* (in response to "Who's wearing your hat?"); contractible copula (e.g., *man's big, man is big*); contractible auxiliary (e.g., *daddy's drinking juice; daddy is drinking juice*)

Source: Adapted from Owens, 2008.

aspects of language development for children 12 through 36 months, are included in **Table 2–3.** By age 3 years, the typically developing child uses utterances two to three words in length, longer verb forms (e.g., *gotta, hafta, gonna*), contractions (e.g., *can't, don't*), regular past tense *-ed*, plurals, and possessives.

Table 2–3 Milestones of Language Development in Toddlers (12 Through 36 Months)

Age	Form		Content	Use
	Phonology	Syntax and Morphology	Semantics	Pragmatics Locutionary Stage (~12+)
12 Months	Unintelligible speech mostly (except for a few words)	Half of all utterances are single nouns	Produce first word	Use referential gestures (e.g., waving hand for "bye-bye"); use line of regard, gestures, voice direction, and body posture to infer intention of others' actions
16 Months	Intelligibility (25% of all words)	One-third of all utterances are single nouns; use negation (*no*); MLU of ~1.31; in Brown's Stage 1	Produce between 3 and 20 words	Engage in verbal turn taking
20 Months	Spoken words processed incrementally	MLU of 1.62; begin to use grammatical morphemes (e.g., -*ing*)	Produce ~50 words (by 18 mos.). Use some verbs and adjectives	Use combinations of words and gestures or two gestures

(continued)

Table 2–3 (Continued)

Age	Form Phonology	Form Syntax and Morphology	Content Semantics	Use Pragmatics Locutionary Stage (~12+)
24 Months	Intelligibility (65% of all words); use rising intonation to ask questions	Use two-word combinations; use prepositions (e.g., in, on); use plural and possessive morphemes, use some irregular past tense verbs; MLU of ~1.92; in Brown's Stage II	Produce ~200 words; understand ~500 words	Use imaginative, heuristic, and informative language functions
28 Months	Intelligibility (70% of all words); phonological processes evident (e.g., final consonant deletion, substitution of consonants)	In Brown's Stage III; mastery of present progressive morpheme (i.e., ing)	Overgeneralize (i.e., extend) one-third of all new words; attend to sentence structure when learning new words	Introduce and change topics of conversation; engage in short dialogues
32 up to 36 Months	Intelligibility (80% of all words); most phonological processes suppressed	One-fourth of all utterances are single nouns and one-fourth are single verbs; MLU ~2.85–3.16; use contractions	Produce ~500 words; understand ~900 words; ask simple questions	Can clarify and request clarification in conversations

Source: Adapted from Owens, 2008; Pence & Justice, 2008.

Milestones of Language Development in the Preschool-Age Child from 3 Through 5 Years (36–60 Months)

Form (Phonology, Morphology, Syntax)

Language development in the preschool-age child is characterized by explosive growth and refinement of all language components. The most important change occurs, however, in language form (syntax, morphology, and phonology). Advances in morphological development are greatest in children between 4 and 7 years old (Owens, 2008). As previously mentioned, utterance length begins as a single morpheme (or word) and increases throughout this period. Additional grammatical morphemes, such as verb endings, appear and are mastered. As sentence complexity also expands, the child's MLU lengthens accordingly (see **Table 2–4**).

By the end of preschool, the child has mastered most adult syntax and morphology. The complexity of forms children produce is surprising considering the short time they have had for acquisition. By age 5 years, the child produces all of the following and more: contractions (e.g., *didn't, doesn't*), modal auxiliaries (e.g., *would, wouldn't, could, couldn't*), various complex forms of the copula and auxiliary "to be" (e.g., *isn't, aren't, weren't, wasn't*), tag questions (e.g., *She's coming too, OK?*), and relative clauses embedded into the object position of the sentence (e.g., *That's the doll that I took*). The following selected example illustrates the increasing complexity in sentence form evident during this period. At 37 months, a child produces embedded infinitive phrases, such as *I'm gonna clean my room up*. By 60 months, the child will produce an embedded infinitive phrase within a relative clause: *There's nothing else I do to help my friend*.

Content (Semantics)

From Chapter 1, we learned that semantics relates to the meaningful use of language across many levels: in isolated words, in sentences, and in larger contexts, including conversation and narratives. At the word level, the growth in semantics is evident in the preschool-age child. For example, whereas the toddler at 2 years old has an expressive vocabulary of about 200 words, the 3-year-old is reported to have a vocabulary of around 1,000 words and uses on average 12,000 words per day (Owens, 2008). By age 5 years, the child understands between 2,500 and 2,800 words and uses between 1,500 and 2,200 of these expressively. In

Table 2–4 Milestones of Language Development in Preschoolers (3 Through 5 Years; 36 Through 60 Months)

Age	Form			Content	Use
	Phonology	Syntax and Morphology	Semantics		Pragmatics
36 Months (3 Years)	Begin to develop shallow phonological awareness	3–5-word sentences; form compound sentences w/conjunction *and*	Use pronouns (e.g., *they, them, us*); fast mapping still used to learn new words Produce 900–1,000 words; follows two-step commands		Engage in longer dialogues
40 Months	Refine articulation	Use pronouns consistently; use adverbs of time	Produce 1,000–1,500 words Understand 1,500–2,000 words Some relational terms understood (e.g., hard–soft)		Use primitive narratives; make limited conversational repairs
44 Months	Most consonants mastered	Use articles (e.g., *a, the*); use past tense and contractions consistently	Some kinship terms understood; syntactic information used to understand meaning of new words		Understand indirect requests when accompanied by pointing
48 Months (4 years)	Reduced use of phonological processes (e.g., weak-syllable deletion, cluster reduction)	4–7-word sentences; use both contractible and uncontractible auxiliaries; use irregular third person verbs (e.g., *has*)	Produces 1,500 words, over-extension of new words via object function; animacy information used to understand meaning of new words; reflexive pronouns used (e.g., *himself, herself, itself*)		Use interpretive, logical, participatory, and organizing functions; construct true narrative

52 Months	Intelligibility good in connected speech; most consonants mastered (but not in every context)	Use both coordination and subordination in sentences; consistently use irregular plural forms	Produce questions using *what* (e.g., *what do, what does, what did*)	Produce indirect requests
56–60 Months (5 Years)	Knows letters of own name; difficulty w/ only later-developing sounds; some phonological processes persist (e.g., liquid gliding, substitution)	5–8-word sentences	Produce 1,500–2,200 words; Understand 2,500–2,800 words; Use deictic terms: *this, that, here, there*; Can follow three-step commands	Use narrative with event sequence but no main character or theme

Source: Adapted from Owens, 2008; Pence & Justice, 2008.

summary, between 3 and 5 years, the child's vocabulary has doubled, and between 2 and 5 years, it has increased 10-fold.

Within sentences, meanings expressed by 2-year-olds include coordination, sequence, and causality, among others. However, as children age, they add additional relational meanings, and those children between 3 and 4 years are able to express temporal sequences (e.g., *I will draw a star after I finish this*), as well as conditionality (e.g., *I wear this while walking*) (Bernstein & Levey, 2009).

Children progress in both comprehension and expression of meaning in larger discourse genres at the same time. For example, in narratives, meaning results from not only sentences composed of individual words but also in the relationship between these sentences. They collectively form a gestalt to communicate a story or an event that is larger than the sum of its parts (i.e., the individual words and sentences). Narratives begin to develop in the preschool years and continue into the elementary school age and beyond. Narratives seen in 3-year-olds are first organized as heaps (i.e., unrelated information) and then by chaining, in which items are grouped together but in no particular order. By 4 years, however, children produce better-organized narratives, in which the elements are focused on a central theme.

In summary, the semantic development of preschoolers reflects growth in lexical (i.e., word) meaning, relational meaning (i.e., meaning between referents reflected in sentences), and contextual meaning (i.e., meaning driven by the context that supports understanding across sentences).

Use (Pragmatics)

Preschool children refine their developing language skills primarily within the context of conversation that initially occurs with the primary caregiver and other family members. Children learn a myriad of polite forms (e.g., *please, thank you, excuse me*), greetings, ways to ask questions and express dissatisfaction and pleasure, and many other forms for communicating that are appropriate to the context and to their communication partner. By age 3, many children have become chatty and introduce topics and maintain conversational turns over several exchanges. By 5 years, about half of all children are able to sustain a topic for more than a dozen turns (Owens, 2008).

In addition to developing longer conversational turns, the preschooler becomes increasingly adept at perspective taking. This is evidenced by the

4-year-old's use of child-directed speech (i.e., motherese) with younger children. Preschoolers also are able to change the form of requests, depending on the perceived status of their conversational partner.

In summary, conversational skills continue to develop in the 3- to 5-year-old and are increasingly adult-like. Children learn to produce indirect requests and to demonstrate more tact and awareness of their conversational partners. They are increasingly able to maintain topics of conversation and to use different registers and forms of speech according to the conversational context.

Milestones of Language Development in School-Age Children

Children enter school with an impressive command of language form. Most produce all phonemes and major syntactic constructions correctly. Nevertheless, growth in both form and content continues. More complex syntactic structures are added or mastered, new words are learned, and meanings of previously learned words are refined.

A key area of growth during the school-age years occurs in pragmatics, as the child increasingly understands how language may be used. School instruction frequently employs **decontextualized language** (i.e., language that is not tied to the here and now) (Berko Gleason, 2009). Accordingly, children must acquire additional knowledge, skills, and strategies to learn and process such language. Knowledge of how language is used in turn influences the child's choice of words and the form the message takes. Major language developments during the school-age years include the elaboration of discourse and growth of **metalinguistic ability**. Metalinguistics refers to the ability to reflect on language as an entity and to analyze it. This ability is instrumental for acquiring literacy, which occurs during the school years. Descriptions of changes in language form, content, and use, as well as an overview of the development of literacy in children (ages 6 through 18 years) follow (see **Table 2–5**).

Form (Phonology, Morphology, Syntax)

The decontextualized language of school instruction requires children to enhance their understanding and use of language. Changes in language form evident in school-age children include the appearance of additional morphemes, use of more complex syntax, and refined usage of nouns and verbs.

Table 2–5 Milestones of Language Development in School-Aged Children Across Domains/Modalities

| Age | Oral (Speech/Listening) | | | | | Written (Reading/Writing/Spelling) |
| | Form | | Content | | Use | |
	Phonology	Morphology and Syntax	Semantics		Pragmatics	
5–6 Years	Mastery of morphophonemic rules re: plural *s* (e.g., /s/ vs. /z/ vs. /ɪz/; can blend and segment sounds and manipulate phonemes in words	Passives understood; morphology beginning to be used to infer meaning of new words; use of sentences that are both more complex syntactically and correctly formulated	Beginning use of multiword (vs. single-word) definitions; expressive vocabulary of 2,600 words and 20,000–24,000 understood		Mostly direct requests used; repetition used for conversational repair; production of minimally four types of narratives	Learning to read by decoding (identifies sounds for printed letters and synthesizes across letters); learns some sight words and conventional spelling for some words; writing more simple than speech
7–8 Years	Production of all sounds and blends (American English)	Derivational suffixes used (e.g., *-er, -ist, -y, -ly*); some passives, elaborated noun phrases, adverbs, conjunctions, and some mental and linguistic verbs used; understand conjunctions (e.g., *because, so, if, but, before, after, then*)	Pronouns used anaphorically (i.e., refer to a previously named noun); word definitions include synonym, categories; words understood to have multiple meanings		Indirect requests and hints understood; most deictic terms understood and used; narrative plots produced w/ beginning, end, problem, and resolution	Dictionary used to define new words; decoding skills effective for reading unfamiliar words; learns spelling patterns (e.g., *-ight* pattern words); writing level akin to speech complexity; mixes oral and literate styles in writing

Age					
9–10 Years		Mental and linguistic verbs (e.g., *believe, promise*) used; pronouns referring to elements outside immediate sentence used; reflexive pronouns used (e.g., *herself, himself*); irreversible passives produced (e.g., *the ball was thrown by the boy*)	Vocabulary in school texts increasingly abstract and more specific than that of conversation; students expected to get information from text knows ~40,000 words by 10 years	Topics sustained through many conversational turns; perceived source of conversational breakdowns addressed; all elements of narrative story grammar produced	Reading to learn w/ focus on reading for information; becoming fluent w/ automatic and efficient decoding; writing takes on more literate style w/subordinate clauses
11–12 Years	Expression of precise intent through stress and emphasis	*If* and *though* understood; Reversible passives produced (e.g., *the girl was kissed by the boy*); derivational suffixes mastered by 12 years (i.e., *-ful, -less, -ly, -ness, -al, -ance, -men, -ity, -ify, -ous, -ive*)	Able to create abstract definitions; ~50,000 words understood	Abstract topics of conversation sustained	Reading on a general adult level; reading to expand vocabulary

(continued)

Table 2–5 (Continued)

| Age | Oral (Speech/Listening) | | | | Written (Reading/Writing/Spelling) |
| | Form | Content | Use | | |
	Phonology	Morphology and Syntax	Semantics	Pragmatics	
13–15 Years		*Unless* understood; all types of clausal embedding understood	Some proverbs understood	Jokes w/ lexical and syntactic ambiguities understood	Multiple points of view considered when reading; writing-level complexity begins to exceed that of speech
16–18 Years	Vowel-shifting rules used (i.e., vowel pronunciation varies across word derivations as in: *sane* vs. *sanity*)	More words used per communication unit in written vs. spoken language; increased use of verb tenses w/ perfect aspect (e.g., *I have eaten all the cookies*)	Command of ~60,000 word meanings ~80,000 by 18 years	Sarcasm, double meanings, and metaphors used; multiple perspectives are recognized	

Source: Adapted from McGregor, 2004; Owens, 2008; Paul, 2007; Pence & Justice, 2008.

Morphemes

Additional **derivational morphemes** continue to appear. Derivational morphemes change word meaning when added. For example, at age 7 years, children acquire the morpheme *ist* (e.g., *piano* changes to *pianist* and *organ* changes to *organist*). Other derivational morphemes that emerge in the school years may also change a word's part of speech in addition to its meaning. For example, when *-ful* is added to *thank*, a verb, the result is *thankful*, an adjective. The following **derivational suffixes** are mastered by age 12 years: *-ful, -less, -ly, -ness, -al, -ance, -men, -ity, -ify, -ous, -ive*.

Syntax

Children produce increasingly longer and more complex sentences during the school years. Length and complexity increase because of **conjoining**, **embedding**, and elaborating the noun or verb phrase. An example of a conjoined sentence (i.e., two clauses joined by a **conjunction**) is, *She finished her exam although she was ill*.

Embedding refers to including a clause within a noun or verb phrase of the sentence. Children of school age grow increasingly adept at understanding various types of embedding and consequently in producing them. The progression in understanding embedding follows: (1) parallel center embedding in which that same subject (i.e., *girl*) serves both clauses (e.g., *The girl who bought the dress went to the party*); (2) parallel ending embedding in which the same object (i.e., *gift*) serves both clauses (e.g., *He gave me a gift that I don't like*), (3) nonparallel ending embedding in which the object (i.e., *boy*) of the main clause is the subject of the embedded clause (e.g., *She hit the boy who ran away*), and (4) nonparallel center embedding in which the subject of the main clause (i.e., *cat*) is the object of the embedded one (e.g., *The cat that was chased by the dog ran up a tree*).

Noun or verb phrase elaboration occurs by adding modifiers. For example, elaboration of the noun phrase in *he wanted to buy the bike* becomes *he wanted to buy the <u>bright</u>, <u>shiny</u>, <u>new</u> bike* by adding numerous descriptive adjectives (i.e., *bright, shiny, new*). Likewise, elaboration of the verb phrase occurs by adding modifiers (e.g., adverbs or adverbial phrases). In addition, passive forms are mastered during the school years.

Content (Semantics)

Growth in semantics results from an increase in the number of words understood and used, as well as elaboration and refinement of meanings of words already within the child's lexicon. Because of the school environment in which increasingly decontextualized language is used, the child develops more richly elaborated meanings, including nondominant and nonliteral (i.e., figurative) word meanings (McGregor, 2004). The expansion of children's figurative language is evident in their use of humor and abstract linguistic forms (simile, metaphor, idioms, and proverbs).

Vocabulary development in school-age children continues to expand at a rate of approximately 3,000 words per year (Just & Carpenter, 1987). For example, a 10-year-old child knows 40,000 words, whereas an 18-year-old knows nearly 80,000 words (see Table 2–5). Comprehension continues to exceed production at every age.

In particular, through the school years with repeated exposure to words, children's word meanings are more precise and increasingly more complex. Semantic development is enhanced as children expand their communication from conversation to narrative and oral and written expository discourse.

Semantic networks, whose development begins around 2 years, continue to be expanded and refined in school-age children, with a shift from syntagmatic (i.e., thematic) to paradigmatic (i.e., taxonomic) associations. For example, in word association tasks, the word *car* might elicit the response *drives* from a 5-year-old following a syntactic progression, where *car* would elicit the response *truck* in a 9-year-old who provides a word of the same "class," or "paradigm." The school-age child increasingly thinks abstractly and may use figurative or nonliteral language. This is apparent in the child's increasing ability to use the following forms: similes and metaphors, idioms, proverbs, and humor.

Use (Pragmatics)

Conversational skills continue to improve during the school years with enhanced repair strategies and increased sensitivity to the conversational partner. The ability to consider multiple perspectives at the same time (i.e., decentration) emerges. In addition, the development of narrative skills continues with story elements (i.e., story grammar), which becomes increasingly complex and more complete. Skills improve in other genres, and the child is required to produce expository speech to fulfill educational assignments. Language growth occurs across modalities as the child becomes increasingly effective in reading and writing.

Literacy

During the school years, the development of metalinguistic skills enables the child to learn to read and write. Initially, the child uses phonemic awareness skills to "crack" the linguistic code. Applying the alphabetic principle (i.e., sound-letter correspondence) and decoding characterize early stages of reading. Around 9 years, the child passes from the learning to read stage into the reading to learn stage, where reading becomes automatic. The focus is now on comprehension as the child reads increasingly in various subject areas. The mastery of language in another modality (i.e., reading and writing) fosters the ongoing and continuous development of word and world knowledge. A reciprocal relationship truly exists between oral and written language wherein learning taking place in one modality informs knowledge in the other.

It is beyond the scope of this chapter to detail all the specific syntactic forms acquired as language develops. The interested reader is encouraged to explore various references cited for additional information. Judith Johnston's "The Chart" is highly recommended when considering intervention targets based on typical language development (Johnston, 2007).

Chapter Summary

For heuristic purposes, language acquisition in the typically developing child is divided into three distinct periods: (1) birth to 2 years, (2) the preschool years (ages 3 through 5 years), and (3) the school years. At birth, infants communicate their needs on a reflexive basis by reacting to internal states and environmental stimulation. Initially, this communication is unintentional and nonspecific. Adult caregivers interpret and assign meaning to these generalized reactions and provide for the baby's needs. During the first year of life, the infant first uses gestures and then words to indicate specific wants and needs. By age 2 years, children are using words and simple word combinations to convey various messages. By the time children enter school, their language has increased dramatically. They use elaborate sentence structures, and others can readily understand them. During the school years, language continues to develop, but not as dramatically as in the preschool years. Impressive gains are seen, however, in the social use of language, reflecting the child's cognitive development and social maturation. The influence of the classroom and peers becomes increasingly important as the child spends fewer hours each day at home with family members and more time in school classrooms and with classmates. In addition, literacy has a major positive effect on language development for all children.

Terms from the Chapter

Conjoining *(27)*
Conjunction *(27)*
Decontextualized language *(23)*
Derivational morphemes *(27)*
Derivational suffixes *(27)*
Embedding *(27)*
Grammatical morpheme *(13)*
Illocutionary *(12)*

Joint reference *(12)*
Locutionary *(12)*
Mean length of utterance *(13)*
Metalinguistic ability *(23)*
Overextension *(13)*
Perlocutionary *(12)*
Underextension *(13)*

References

Berko Gleason, J. (2009). The development of language: An overview and a preview. In J. Berko Gleason & N. Bernstein Ratner (Eds.), *The development of language* (7th ed., pp. 1–36). Boston, MA: Pearson.

Bernstein, D. K., & Levey, S. (2009). Language development: A review. In D. K. Bernstein & E. Tiegerman-Farber (Eds.), *Language and communication disorders in children* (6th ed., pp. 28–100). Boston, MA: Pearson.

Denes, P. B., & Pinson, E. N. (1993). *The speech chain: The physics and biology of spoken language.* New York, NY: W. H. Freeman.

Haynes, W. O., & Shulman, B. B. (1994). *Communication development: Foundations, processes, and clinical applications.* Englewood Cliffs, NJ: Prentice Hall.

Hegde, M. N. (2001). *Introduction to communication disorders* (3rd ed.). Austin, TX: PRO-ED.

Johnston, J. (2007). *Thinking about language.* Greenville, SC: Thinking Publications.

Just, M. A., & Carpenter, P. A. (1987). *The psychology of reading and language comprehension.* Boston, MA: Allyn and Bacon.

McGregor, K. (2004). Developmental dependencies between lexical semantics and reading. In C. A. Stone, E. R. Silliman, B. J. Ehren, & K. Apel (Eds.), *Handbook of language & literacy: Development and disorders* (pp. 302–317). New York, NY: Guilford Press.

Owens, R. E. (2008). *Language development* (7th ed). Boston, MA: Pearson.

Paul, R. (2007). *Language disorders from infancy through adolescence* (3rd ed). St. Louis, MO: Mosby.

Pence, K. L., & Justice, L. M. (2008). *Language development from theory to practice*. Upper Saddle River, NJ: Pearson.

Piaget, J. (1954). *The construction of reality in the child*. New York: Basic Books.

Pinker, S. (1984). *Language learnability and language development*. Cambridge, MA: Harvard University Press.

C H A P T E R   3

Language Disorders in Children

Bill Cupples

Chapter Objectives

After reading this chapter, you should be able to:

- Describe the questions to be answered to determine the presence of a language disorder.
- Describe the terms used to define the diagnostic categories of language disorders.
- Describe two methods for classifying language disorders.
- Describe the advantages and disadvantages of using the two systems.

Definitions

The term **language disorders** encompasses a broad range of language and learning differences found in children with a variety of diagnoses. The American Speech-Language-Hearing Association (ASHA) has described language disorders as deficits in "impaired comprehension and/or use of spoken, written and/or other symbol systems. This disorder may involve (1) the form of language (phonology, morphology, syntax), (2) the content of language (semantics), and/or (3) the function of language in communication (pragmatics) in any combination" (ASHA, 1993, p. 30). On the basis of this definition, a number of questions need to be answered to determine whether a given child possesses a language disorder:

- Is there impaired comprehension/understanding of spoken language?
- Is there impaired use of expressive spoken language (talking)?
- Is there impaired comprehension of written language (reading comprehension)?

- Is there impaired use of expressive written language (reading aloud, writing)?
- Is there impaired comprehension/understanding of the form of language?
- Is there impaired use/expression of the form of language?
- Is there impaired comprehension/understanding of the content of language?
- Is there impaired use/expression of the content of language?
- Is there impaired comprehension/understanding of the **pragmatics** of language?
- Is there impaired use/expression of the pragmatics of language?

We will discuss these questions more fully in the chapter on assessing language disorders.

Deficits in **language form** represent difficulties children might have in comprehending and producing the rules that govern how we create sentences, including syntax or grammar; morphological features, such as affixes to mark plurals, possession, and negation; and rules that govern the way sounds/phonemes can be combined in a language to represent a word. Deficits in **language content** describe the difficulties some children have in using the vocabulary/lexicon of a language, and in determining how categories of words are related to each other. Deficits in **language use**, or pragmatics, occur when a child does not understand the social rules of communication that change depending on the context and purpose of communication, the status of the participants in the conversation, and the genre (Bloom & Lahey, 1978).

Many terms have been used to describe the learning differences associated with language disorders. These terms include **childhood aphasia** (Eisenson & Ingram, 1972), **language deviance**, **language delay**, and **specific language impairment (SLI)** (Paul, 2007). Although there are some children with language differences due to a neurological disorder, aphasia more accurately describes the language impairments observed in adults following a stroke (Davis, 2007). Recent research has revealed a genetic component in some children with these language differences that further implies that aphasia is not the most descriptive term (Tomblin, 2008). More recently, researchers and practitioners in the fields associated with language disorders have begun using the term **language impairment** to describe the behaviors we have discussed. Paul (2007) states that the use of the term **impairment** is more neutral. We often think of a *disorder* as a medical or physiological condition, thus denoting some kind of physical illness.

Disorder also implies some kind of difference in how these children learn, when, in reality, most of the children in this population exhibit similar learning patterns to those in typically developing children (Norbury, Tomblin & Bishop, 2008). **Language deviance** has strong connotations of irregular or unusual behaviors, beyond what would be considered acceptable in the typical population. Although some children in this population exhibit unusual behaviors, they also exhibit typical behaviors of growing and developing children, thus they are not really children with deviant learning patterns. Impairment simply indicates that something is different about a child's learning style and avoids the negative connotations of the word **disorder**. Impairment also fits well with the World Health Organization's (WHO) continuum of the effect of an impairment on an individual. The impairment is the physical or structural difference a person is experiencing; the **activity** is the effect the impairment has on a person's activities of daily living and interaction with the environment, including the way the person views his or her impairment and chooses to adapt to the impairment. **Participation** looks at the social consequences of the impairment, to what extent social, political, and cultural attitudes and policies promote or inhibit a person's ability to experience society to the fullest (Rosenbaum & Stewart, 2004). Specific language impairment is used to describe children whose deficits are restricted to **language comprehension** and expression, with other abilities developing roughly within the typical range of development (Norbury et al., 2008). In this book, we will use language disorders and language impairment interchangeably.

Descriptions of Language Impairments: Etiologic-Based Models

Language impairments in children have generally been described either by using an etiologic-based classification system or a descriptively based one. The etiologic-based system assumes that children within a specific causative group have similar language and learning abilities. Some of the etiologic categories discussed in the literature follow:

- Cognitive impairment
- Language-based learning disability
- Autism spectrum disorder
- Hearing impairment
- Traumatic brain injury
- Genetic and chromosomal disorder
- Specific language impairment

In children with **cognitive impairment (CI)** the assumption is that their intellectual abilities, as assessed by appropriate standardized tests, are roughly 1.5 to 2 standard deviations below the mean intelligence levels of their age-matched peers. With a mean or average **intelligence quotient (IQ)** of 100 and a standard deviation of 15, we expect that children in the cognitive impairment category will have IQs of 75 or lower (Bloom & Lahey, 1978). We also assume that language learning will be influenced by the degree of cognitive impairment. Children with IQs of 60 to 75, for example, will be able to learn more language concepts than children with IQs below 60. We assume that all children in this category will have language impairments because of a decreased ability to process auditory information, to remember information they have heard, to attend to information, and to generalize information they experience. Children with cognitive impairment usually need many examples of a concept to acquire the full understanding of the concept.

In children with a **language-based learning disability (LLD)**, we assume that at least some of their cognitive abilities are within the typical range of development when their IQ is compared with their age-matched peers. These children have differences restricted to learning language that may also extend to reading and writing deficits. The learning profiles of these children will vary, depending on the specific nature of the profile of strengths and needs (Paul, 2007). Thus, a careful differential diagnosis of these children is required to determine the specific needs to be addressed. We will further discuss assessment and diagnosis in Chapter 4 ("Assessment of Child Language Disorders").

In children with **autism spectrum disorder (ASD)**, we see particular differences in language learning and use related to stereotypic behavior patterns, insistence on sameness, and difficulties in communication, leading to difficulties in navigating social interaction. These children exhibit a range of cognitive abilities. Some will be verbal, while others may be nonverbal or require some augmentative or alternative communication system. The common variables in these differences relate to the stereotypic behavior patterns, insistence on sameness, and difficulty in social interaction. Many of these children are visual learners. Because of these visual strengths, visual supports, such as pictures to communicate or visual schedules of the activities of the day, may be used to keep them oriented to the context and attending to the planned activities (Hall, 2009).

Hearing impairment can arise from various etiologies. The significant feature in hearing impairment is that children lack the auditory abilities to be able to acquire language in a typical fashion. Because most children with hearing impairment possess intelligence in the typical range, the major learning challenge is to have appropriate amplification through hearing aids or cochlear implants or to acquire another language system to communicate, such as sign language. Given the absence of other developmental factors, when these issues are resolved, we expect that these children will begin to acquire language and to communicate as children who develop typically.

Children with **traumatic brain injury (TBI)** typically experience the usual developmental sequences of language and communication until they sustain some kind of neurologic damage. This damage usually occurs from a closed-head injury, such as an automobile accident or a fall, or from an external insult such as a gunshot wound. Depending on the degree of damage, they may recover full language functioning, may experience subtle cognitive deficits, such as planning difficulties and memory deficits, or may have severe enough damage that communication will occur with an alternative/augmentative communication system. They may also possess various forms of learning disabilities depending on the location and extent of the damage (Ylvisaker, 1998).

Some recent research focuses on the effect of genetics on language impairments. On the basis of research advances, we know a component of genetic transmission can be found in some children with language impairments, including children with learning disabilities and autism. Some researchers now believe that genetics is a factor in the majority of language impairments. Linkages to SLI have been found on chromosomes 16 and 19, among others (Newbury & Monaco, 2008). In addition to these recent genetic studies investigating the heritability of language impairments, we also know of particular types of language impairment related to specific genetic syndromes. Some examples of genetic-based syndromes that present with cognitive and language impairments include **Down syndrome**, **Prader-Willi syndrome**, **Rett syndrome** (currently on the autism spectrum) Williams syndrome, and **fragile X syndrome** (McDuffie & Abbeduto, 2008).

As stated earlier, children with SLI, much like language-based learning disabilities, are believed to have deficits restricted to comprehending and expressing language. These children will have intelligence in the typical range, as measured by IQ scores, compared with their age-matched peers but will have marked difficulties in learning language form, content, or use (Norbury et al., 2008). Within this category are young children who exhibit delays in using expressive language but whose language comprehension and development in other areas appear to be typical. These children have been referred to as late talkers (Rescorla & Roberts, 2002).

Here are two of the difficulties with using the etiologic-based models to describe language impairments: (1) We assume that each category is relatively discrete, that the children who fall within a particular category are *alike* in some crucial ways, and *not like* children in the other categories in some crucial ways. (2) We use measures of intelligence to sort out discrete abilities, and then use those measures to assign a given child to a particular category.

1. *The distinctness of the categories*: Research has demonstrated that children within each etiologic category are not always like all the other children in that category and that children across etiologic categories may share similar abilities (Johnston, 2006). A wide range of abilities and learning patterns are represented in each category of CI, LLD, ASD, TBI, **genetic and chromosomal disorders**, and SLI. Even though there are some similarities within each etiologic category, practitioners have found that, for children within each diagnostic category, it is important to plan intervention goals and objectives for each child as an individual, based on their individual learning styles, and not based on the etiologic category to which a child is assigned (Owens, 2006). Research in the area of LLD has demonstrated similarities in the learning patterns of children with SLI and children diagnosed with LLD (Owens, 2006). Research in ASD has demonstrated that the learning patterns and profiles of children with ASD overlap in some ways with the learning patterns and profiles of children with SLI (Bishop, 2008). Thus, the etiologic categories turn out to be formal theoretic constructs with little evidence to support that they are discrete categories in actual practice.
2. *Use of intelligence measures*: Many of these categories use intelligence, as measured by IQ scores, to determine whether a child fits within a given category. This practice is called **cognitive referencing** (Cole, 2007; McCauley, 2001). Cognitive referencing has some pitfalls. Some of the difficulties noted with cognitive referencing are as follows:

    -   Cultural and linguistic biases in test construction, administration, and scoring
    -   The assumption that some tests assess nonverbal intelligence as a separate intelligence from verbal (language) intelligence

- The assumption that IQ is a static measurement not subject to change

Most of the tests used to assess intelligence and learning patterns in children possess some form of cultural and linguistic bias. The children in the normative samples used to develop the administration and scoring procedures for the test may represent linguistic and cultural populations that differ from the child who is taking the test. In addition, many of our tests use normative samples of typical children to develop the administration and scoring procedures, while we use the test to assess the abilities of children we believe to be atypical learners. Thus, we are using an assessment procedure that was not developed to consider the specific atypical learning patterns of a given child.

Many of these tests assume that it is possible to assess nonverbal abilities as a separate entity from verbal abilities. In fact, nonverbal tests often use language for directions or instructions to describe what a child has to do to complete the test. Thus, a child with language comprehension deficits will be penalized on the test because he or she does not understand the directions adequately to complete the test. Research has also demonstrated that language abilities are often used in problem-solving tasks that appear to be nonverbal. Children with better language abilities will be able to complete the nonverbal task more accurately because they use internal verbal mediation to solve the problem. It appears, then, that we cannot always assess nonverbal intelligence as a discrete set of abilities separate from verbal intelligence. Therefore, cognitive referencing may not be the appropriate way to assign a child to a particular etiologic category.

Cognitive referencing also assumes that a child's IQ is a stable constant, so that placement and planning can be based on this stable measure of intelligence. We now know that IQ is not a stable measure, and thus, our assumptions about a diagnostic category based on cognitive referencing are false (McCauley, 2001).

Clinicians often have to use the etiologic-based models because the diagnostic categories derived from these models are used to determine eligibility for speech and language services. State departments of education often require school clinicians to select one or more diagnostic categories on the **individualized education plan** to establish that a child should receive their services. Many third-party reimbursers (Medicaid, insurance companies) require a particular diagnosis before the services are reimbursed.

Descriptions of Language Impairments: Descriptively Based Models

The descriptively based system views language disorders as representing deficiencies along one or more of the linguistic parameters as compared with chronologic-age-based expectations. In the descriptively based systems, we are more interested in ascertaining the learning and developmental profile of each child as an individual using a prescribed set of parameters, rather than trying to determine the particular etiologic category for a child. We have already discussed some concepts crucial to the descriptively based models. In this model, it is important to determine the developmental profile of a child based on language form, content, and use.

The questions we posed at the beginning of the chapter need to be investigated if we are to describe the language impairment in each child from this perspective. We need to determine, as specifically as possible, the relationship of a child's language comprehension (receptive language) to his or her expressive language. In addition, receptive and expressive language needs to be investigated in each of the areas of language form, content, and use (Bloom & Lahey, 1978, Owens, 2006). There are several advantages to using the descriptively based system over the etiologically based one. The first advantage is that an individual profile of abilities and learning style is developed for each child. We make no assumptions about a child's abilities or learning styles based on the diagnosis, but, rather, after a careful look at all of a child's language abilities. The second advantage is that the profile we develop gives us information to write more specific goals and objectives for each individual child (Paul, 2007). We will discuss these issues in detail in Chapter 4 ("Assessment of Child Language Disorders"), Chapter 5 ("Intervention Goals"), and Chapter 6 ("Approaches to Intervention").

Prevalence of Language Impairments

Prevalence is defined as the number of people who have a particular disorder or impairment at any given time. It is difficult to describe the exact prevalence of language impairments. Prevalence depends on which term is used to describe the impairment because of the overlap of characteristics of language impairment across diagnostic categories and because of **comorbidity** across diagnostic categories. Comorbidity refers to the occurrence of more than one impairment or medical diagnosis within a diagnostic category. For instance, children with LLD may have attention deficit disorders as a comorbid diagnosis. Children with ASD may have diagnoses of seizure disorder or **tuberous sclerosis** as a comorbid diagnosis.

If we look at ASD as a category, for example, the prevalence rates are about 150 for every 1,000 births (Counting Autism, 2009). This rate does not include other impairments we would classify as language impairments. If we look at language disorders as a whole, some sources suggest a prevalence of 8 to 12 percent in the preschool years (Child Language Disorders, 2009). This is believed to fall to 2 to 8 percent by early elementary school (Feldman, 2005).

Chapter Summary

Language impairment describes a variety of children with a variety of educational profiles and diagnostic labels. Children with language impairments may have difficulties understanding spoken or written language, expressing themselves with spoken or written language, and understanding and using the rules of social interaction and conversation. There are different models for defining and diagnosing language impairments. Etiologic-based models attempt to determine the kind and degree of language impairment by assessing to obtain an educational or medical diagnosis. Examples of diagnostic categories are cognitive impairment, language-based learning disability, autism spectrum disorder, hearing impairment, traumatic brain injury, genetic and chromosomal disorders, and specific language impairment. Etiologic-based models have two problems: first, abilities of children in each category are not discrete; children across diagnostic categories may present with similar profiles and abilities. Second, cognitive referencing is often used to determine the diagnostic category, even though problems with cognitive referencing have been cited in the literature. Descriptively based models attempt to define a child's abilities by assessing to determine functioning in a variety of language areas, form, content, and use and in the relationship between language comprehension versus language expression. Descriptively based models allow us to develop profiles of abilities for individual children regardless of the diagnostic category and to design individualized intervention programs based on the profile of abilities. The prevalence of language impairments in the general population is difficult to determine, but recent estimates reveal that 8 to 12 percent of preschool children present with language impairments. In school-aged children the figure drops somewhat to 2 to 8 percent.

Terms from the Chapter

Activity *(35)*
Autism spectrum disorder *(36)*
Childhood aphasia *(34)*
Cognitive impairment *(36)*
Cognitive referencing *(38)*
Comorbidity *(40)*
Disorder (35)
Down syndrome *(37)*
Fragile X syndrome *(37)*
Genetic and chromosomal disorder *(38)*
Hearing impairment *(36)*
Impairment *(34)*
Individualized education plan *(39)*
Intelligence quotient *(36)*
Language-based learning disability *(36)*
Language comprehension *(35)*

Language content *(34)*
Language delay *(34)*
Language deviance *(34)*
Language disorder *(33)*
Language form *(34)*
Language impairment *(34)*
Language use *(34)*
Participation *(35)*
Prader-Willi syndrome *(37)*
Pragmatics *(34)*
Prevalence *(40)*
Rett syndrome *(37)*
Specific language impairment (SLI) *(34)*
Traumatic brain injury *(37)*
Tuberous sclerosis *(41)*

References

American Speech-Language-Hearing Association. (1993). Ad Hoc Committee on Service Delivery in the Schools. Rockville, MD: ASHA Reports.

Bishop, D. V. M. (2008). Specific language impairment, dyslexia, and autism: Using genetics to unravel their relationship. In C. F. Norbury, J. B. Tomblin, & D. V. M. Bishop, (Eds.), *Understanding developmental language disorders* (pp. 67–78). New York, NY: Psychology Press.

Bloom, L., & Lahey, M. (1978). *Language development and language disorders.* New York, NY: Wiley.

Child Language Disorders. (2009). Allyn and Bacon comunications disorders supersite. Retrieved from http://wps.ablongman.com/ab_disorders_supersite/6/1541/394656.cw/index.html

Cole, K. N. (2007). Serving secondary students. In A. Kahmi, J. Masterson, & K. Apel (Eds.), *Clinical decision making in developmental language disorders* (pp 307–322). Baltimore, MD: Paul H. Brookes.

Counting Autism. (2009). CDC's autism and developmental disabilities monitoring network. Retrieved from http://www.cdc.gov/Features/CountingAutism/

Davis, G. A. (2007). *Aphasiology: Disorders and clinical practice* (2nd ed.). Boston, MA: Allyn & Bacon.

Eisenson, J., & Ingram, D. (1972). Childhood aphasia: An updated concept based on recent research. *Papers and Reports on Child Language Development, 4,* 103–120.

Feldman, H. M. (2005). Evaluation and management of language and speech disorders in preschool children. *Pediatrics in Review*, *26*, 131–142.

Hall, L. J. (2009). *Autism spectrum disorders: From theory to practice*. Upper Saddle River, NJ: Merrill.

Johnston, J. (2006). *Thinking about child language: From research to practice*. Eau Claire, WI: Thinking Publications.

McCauley, R. J. (2001). *Assessment of language disorders in children*. Mahwah, NJ: Lawrence Erlbaum.

McDuffie A., & Abbeduto, L. (2008). Language disorders in children with mental retardation of genetic origin: Down syndrome, fragile X syndrome, and Williams syndrome. In R. Schwartz (Ed.), *Handbook of child language disorders* (pp. 44–66). New York, NY: Psychology Press.

Newbury, D. F., & Monaco, A. P. (2008). The application of molecular genetics in the study of developmental language disorder. In C. Norbury, J. B. Tomblin, & D.V.M. Bishop (Eds.), *Understanding developmental language disorders* (pp. 79–92). New York, NY: Psychology Press.

Norbury, C., Tomblin, J. B., & Bishop, D. V. M. (Eds.). (2008). *Understanding developmental language disorders*. New York, NY: Psychology Press.

Owens, R. E. (2006). *Language disorders: A functional approach to assessment and intervention* (4th ed.). Boston, MA: Pearson Education.

Paul, R. (2007). *Language disorders from infancy through adolescence: Assessment and intervention* (3rd ed.). Burlington, MA: Elsevier Science.

Rescorla, L., & Roberts, J. (2002). Nominal versus verbal morpheme use in late talkers at ages 3 and 4. *Journal of Speech, Language, and Hearing Research*, *45*, 1219–1231.

Rosenbaum, P., & Stewart, D. (2004). The World Health Organization international classification of functioning, disability, and health: A model to guide clinical thinking, practice, and research in the field of cerebral palsy. *Seminars in Pediatric Neurology*, *11*(1).

Tomblin, J. B. (2008). Validating diagnostic standards for specific language impairment using adolescent outcomes. In C. Norbury, J. B. Tomblin, & D. V. M. Bishop (Eds.), *Understanding developmental language disorders* (pp. 93–116). New York, NY: Psychology Press.

Ylvisaker, M. (1998). *Traumatic brain injury rehabilitation: Children and adolescents* (2nd ed.). Boston, MA: Butterworth-Heinemann.

CHAPTER 4

Assessment of Child Language Disorders

Bill Cupples

Chapter Objectives

After reading this chapter you should be able to:

- Describe the information gathered to assess to determine a diagnosis and eligibility.
- Discuss how to assess to determine goals and objectives.
- Describe how to assess the validity and reliability of a standardized test.
- Describe how scores are used to interpret performance on a standardized test.
- Describe the limitations of standardized testing.
- Describe various criterion-referenced and authentic assessments.
- Describe how a language sample is obtained and analyzed.
- Describe the types of developmental information obtained by analysis of the language sample.
- Discuss how a mean length of utterance is obtained.
- Discuss the importance of grammatical morphemes.
- Describe some informal procedures in addition to the language sample for eliciting language production in children.
- Discuss the principles of dynamic assessment.
- Discuss the issues inherent in the assessment of young children.
- Describe some of the tests used to assess language and communication in children.

As stated in Chapter 3, there are certain questions that need to be answered to determine the presence of a language disorder. These questions are repeated here:

- Is there impaired comprehension/understanding of spoken language?
- Is there impaired use of expressive spoken language (talking)?
- Is there impaired comprehension of written language (reading comprehension)?
- Is there impaired use of expressive written language (reading aloud, writing)?
- Is there impaired comprehension/understanding of the form of language?
- Is there impaired use/expression of the form of language?
- Is there impaired comprehension/understanding of the content of language?
- Is there impaired use/expression of the content of language?

The purpose of assessment or evaluation is to answer these questions as thoroughly as possible to arrive at an accurate diagnosis. As stated in Chapter 3, the diagnosis is essential to determine whether a child and family are eligible to receive speech and language services. However, the kinds of assessment or evaluation procedures used to determine eligibility do not always provide information with enough accuracy and depth for the clinician to write individualized treatment goals and objectives. In actual clinical practice, the speech-language pathologist (SLP) will obtain some information from the assessment used to diagnose and establish eligibility to determine the intervention and treatment goals and objectives. Usually, a more detailed assessment is needed to obtain enough information to determine which intervention strategies will be used and which goals and objectives will be written to meet the individual needs of a child. In this chapter we will discuss two purposes for assessment: (1) assessment to determine a diagnosis and eligibility, and (2) assessment to determine treatment goals and objectives.

Assessment to Determine a Diagnosis and Eligibility

An assessment to determine a diagnosis and **eligibility** usually obtains the following information (Owens, 2004):

- Case history information (e.g., family, medical, social, educational)
- Information on the prerequisites for speech and language (e.g., normal hearing, normal cognitive skills, normal neuromotor and emotional maturation, normal speech mechanism, as well as a stimulating and nourishing home environment)

- Information regarding the nature and severity of the language disorder
- Family interview
- Assessment of speech, language, and hearing abilities
- Assessment of interaction
- Determination of a **prognosis**

The family or the legal guardian is asked to complete a case history of the child. The case history assembles developmental information regarding the mother's pregnancy, the birth, the child's medical history, family information, and medical history, as well as a thorough report of the child's developmental motor, cognitive, social-emotional, hearing, speech, and language history. If the child is school age, then a history of academic performance is also collected. Assessment procedures for infants, toddlers, and preschoolers are slightly different from the procedures used for school-aged children. Special considerations for assessing infants, toddlers, and preschoolers will be discussed later in this chapter.

The SLP reviews the case history to assist in planning for the evaluation session. Usually, a formal family interview is conducted as a follow-up to the case history review because that review may raise additional questions for the SLP. The family interview is also the time to hear directly from the family or caregivers the nature of their concerns about their child's speech and language development.

The SLP then uses a variety of measures to assess all areas of language comprehension and expression that relate to a child's knowledge of language form (syntax, morphology, and phonology), language content (semantics, vocabulary, and lexicon), and language use (pragmatics and social interaction). Usually, some standardized tests are administered in addition to informal measures of speech, language, and communication. In some states, standardized tests are required to establish eligibility for speech and language services. After the testing is completed, the clinician analyzes and interprets all the data to determine the degree of delay and impairment, to make recommendations for intervention, and to establish a prognosis. The prognosis tells a family what the expected outcome of intervention will be.

Standardized Tests

Standardized tests are instruments that have been developed and normed on a population of typical children. The test is administered to a child in a standardized manner described in the test manual. The uniform test administration procedures ensure that the results of this child's assessment can be compared with the **normative sample** on which the instrument was standardized. Thus, a child can be compared with a population of age-matched typical peers to determine whether she is developing in a similar manner. **Table 4–1** describes some commonly used standardized tests.

The SLP should use certain criteria to determine that the test is adequately designed to assess the particular language features that need to be assessed and that the test is standardized adequately so that the scores accurately reflect a child's true ability. The following criteria are usually considered in evaluating a standardized test:

- *Construct validity*: The degree to which a test is constructed to agree with its theoretical premises: that is, if a test purports to measure language abilities, to what extent do the items used to assess abilities actually reflect language abilities?
- *Content validity*: The degree to which test items are chosen with a clear rationale, test items actually measure the specific behaviors intended by the instrument, and test items within the test measure the same behaviors.
- *Reliability*: The degree to which repeated administrations of the test agree with one another. Test-retest **reliability** means that a given child should perform similarly when the test is readministered. Interobserver reliability is the degree to which two examiners trained to use the test will obtain similar results from a given child.
- *Types of scores obtained*: Are the raw scores obtained on the test convertible to scores that allow comparison with the original normative sample and that allow a determination of the degree of impairment? Generally, the better tests convert raw scores to standard or **scaled scores**. This conversion places a child's performance on a numerical distribution that reflects the abilities of a population of typical children and allows comparison between subtests of a test with other tests. Standard scores and scaled scores should always be reported with a **mean** expected score and the predicted standard deviation expected for the score. For example, if a test has a mean standard score of 100 with a **standard deviation** of 15, then we can predict that child with a score falling between 85 and 115 is within the typical range of development. As stated in Chapter 3, we typically expect that children with a language impairment will obtain scores more than one and a half standard deviations below the mean. A child who obtains a standard score of 70 or lower is determined to be

Table 4–1 Selected Standardized Tests for Assessing Language Comprehension and Expression

Name of Test	Age Ranges Assessed	Domains of Assessment
Preschool Language Scale-4 Author(s): Irla Lee Zimmerman, PhD, Violette G. Steiner, BS, and Roberta Evatt Pond, MA Pearson Assessments 800-627-7271 clinicalcustomersupport @pearson.com	Birth to 6; 11 years	Auditory comprehension and expression, language form and content
Clinical Evaluation of Language Fundamentals-IV Author(s): Eleanor Semel, EdD, Elisabeth H. Wiig, PhD, and Wayne A. Secord, PhD Pearson Assessments 800-627-7271 clinicalcustomersupport @pearson.com	5;0 to 21;0	Language comprehension and expression, language form and content, has a profile and observation scale for evaluating pragmatic abilities
Clinical Evaluation of Language Fundamentals—Preschool-2 Author(s): Eleanor Semel, EdD, Elisabeth H. Wiig, PhD, and Wayne A. Secord, PhD Pearson Assessments 800-627-7271 clinicalcustomersupport @pearson.com	3;0 to 6;0	Language comprehension and expression, language form and content, pragmatics profile
Comprehensive Assessment of Spoken Language Author: Elizabeth Carrow-Woolfolk PRO-ED Inc. 800-897-3202 www.proedinc.com	3;0 to 21;11	Language comprehension and expression, language form and content, structured pragmatic assessment

(continued)

Table 4–1 (Continued)

Name of Test	Age Ranges Assessed	Domains of Assessment
Test of Language Development-4 Primary Authors: Phyllis L. Newcomer and Donald D. Hammill Western Psychological Services 800-648-8857	4;0 to 8;11	Language comprehension and expression, language form and content
Test of Language Development-4 Intermediate Authors: Phyllis L. Newcomer and Donald D. Hammill Western Psychological Services 800-648-8857	8;0 to 17;11	Language comprehension and expression, language form and content
Detroit Test of Learning Aptitude-4 Author: Donald D. Hammill PRO-ED Inc. 800-897-3202 www.proedinc.com	6;0 to 17;0	Language comprehension and expression, language form and content, attention, memory, motor
Illinois Test of Psycholinguistic Abilities-3 Authors: Donald D. Hammill, Nancy Mather, and Rhia Roberts Super Duper Publications 800-277-8737 www.superduperinc.com	5;0 to 12;11	Language comprehension, language form and content, spoken and written
MacArthur-Bates Communicative Development Inventories Larry Fenson, PhD, Virginia A. Marchman, PhD, Donna J. Thal, PhD, Philip S. Dale, PhD, J. Steven Reznick, PhD, and Elizabeth Bates, PhD Paul H. Brookes Publishing Co. 800-638-3775 www.brookespublishing.com	8 to 30 months	Parent inventory reporting on the use of words and gestures and words and sentences

Table 4–1 (Continued)

Name of Test	Age Ranges Assessed	Domains of Assessment
Rossetti Infant-Toddler Language Scale Louis Rossetti Linguisystems 800-776-4332 linguisystems.com	Birth to 3;0	Observation scale and parent report; assesses abilities in areas of interaction/attachment, pragmatics, gesture, play, language comprehension and language expression
Carolina Curriculum for Infants and Toddlers Nancy M. Johnson-Martin, PhD, Susan M. Attermeier, PhD, PT, and Bonnie J. Hacker, MHS, OTR/L Paul H. Brookes Publishing Co. 800-638-3775 www.brookespublishing.com	Birth to 36 months	Criterion-referenced assessment log; Assesses development in areas of personal-social, cognition, cognition/communication, communication, fine motor and gross motor skills

significantly delayed when compared with the normative sample of her age-matched peers.

- *Standard error of measure*: To what extent is the score obtained for a given child a *true* measure of her abilities, or is the score subject to some error of measurement that the score actually does *not* represent the child's abilities?

- *Thoroughness and appropriateness of the standardization sample*: To what extent does the normative sample used in the test reflect the actual demographics of the country in terms of the population assessed? Does the test have enough children at the specified age ranges to reflect a typical population? Does the normative sample of the test have an appropriate number of children from the different geographic regions of the country and from rural, suburban, and urban areas? Does the test's normative sample have appropriate representation of socioeconomic status, race, and gender? How old are the norms of the test?

- *Test sensitivity and test specificity*: To what extent does the test actually discriminate children with language impairments from typical children? In other words, how does it discriminate true positives (children who have a language impairment) from true negatives (children who do not have a language impairment)? Too many false positives (indicating that a child has a language impairment when he or she does not) and false negatives (indicating that a child does *not* have a language impairment when he or she does) means that the test does not possess **validity** (Owens, 2004; Paul, 2007).

- *Hypothetical example*: This example was developed to show how a standardized test might be evaluated and how it might be used to assess the language of a child suspected of having language difficulties. The New Test of Language Comprehension and Expression (NTLCE) claims to assess language comprehension and expression in language form and language content. It has a normative sample of 2,100 children aged 5 to 12 years, with 300 children in each year. The standardization sample matches the U.S. population profile in socioeconomic status, race, gender, and geographic distribution of areas of the country and rural, suburban, and urban areas when compared with the 2000 U.S. census. The test has subtests that assess the understanding of single-word vocabulary, the ability to follow commands, the ability to provide definitions of words, the ability to make judgments using sentences with different syntax, and the ability to imitate sentences. The test also analyzes a spontaneous language sample collected in a conversation for various sentence structures.

In the single-word vocabulary subtest, the examiner presents a series of plates with four pictures on each plate. The examiner then says a word, and the student is instructed to point to the picture that best represents the word.

The examiner assesses the child's ability to follow commands by presenting a group of tiles of different shapes, sizes, and colors. The student is expected to manipulate the tiles based on the examiner's commands (e.g., *Place the large red square to the right of the small blue circle*).

In the defining words subtest, the examiner says a word to the student. The student is then expected to provide a verbal definition of the word.

The ability to make judgments using sentences subtest presents a series of plates with four pictures on each plate. The examiner then says a sentence and the student is expected to point to the picture that best represents the sentence (i.e., *Sally saw her mother putting a coat on him.*).

In the ability to imitate sentences subtest, the examiner reads a series of sentences aloud to the student. The student is expected to repeat each sentence exactly as the examiner read it.

The test has a mean total scaled score of 100 with a standard deviation of 15. Each subtest has a mean total scaled score of 10 with a standard deviation of 3. Good test-retest reliability and interobserver reliability is reported.

On the basis of the criteria used for evaluating a standardized test, would we find the NTLCE to be acceptable as a measure for assessing language abilities? Probably yes, but notice that the description still misses some of the crucial elements we need to evaluate a test successfully. We have no information about validity, error of measurement, or test sensitivity and specificity. We would have to investigate the test further to determine how it meets these criteria. Assume that it does, and we decide that this will be one of the tests we use in our assessment protocol to determine a diagnosis and eligibility for speech and language services. Consider the following case:

A Sample Case

J. is a 9-year-old fourth grader who has been referred for speech and language testing by his classroom teacher. Her concerns are that he appears to have difficulty following directions in class and that he does not participate in class discussion. When he presents an oral report he exhibits numerous grammatical errors and has difficulty expressing his thoughts logically and coherently. She states that he "sometimes appears to be talking in circles." A full speech and language evaluation is completed on J. that includes the following:

- *A hearing screening*
- *Oral mechanism examination*
- *Speech screening*
- *Standardized test of vocabulary*
- *A spontaneous language sample collected in an informal conversation with J.*
- *The NTLCE (Note that this is a hypothetical example. We may want to do more standardized testing, depending on the profile obtained from testing a particular child).*

In addition, some informal assessments including a classroom observation, assessment of J.'s abilities using the fourth-grade benchmarks, and informal assessment of J.s understanding of vocabulary from his language arts, social studies, and science texts. Testing indicates that J. has delays in his language abilities, particularly in vocabulary expression, auditory memory, and expressive language. His scores on the NTLCE are as follows:

Single-word vocabulary	*standard score of 8*
Memory for commands	*standard score of 5*
Defining words	*standard score of 4*
Making judgments with syntax	*standard score of 5*
Making a sentence	*standard score of 5*
Sentence imitation	*standard score of 8*

(Mean scaled score = 10, standard deviation = 3)

Analysis of the language sample reveals that J. has difficulty with subject-verb agreement and speaks mostly in simple sentences. His use of compound sentences is limited to and to conjoin subjects, predicates, and series of sentences. No complex sentences were observed in the sample. He has false starts in his sample, indicating that he will start a sentence, stop, and reformulate what he wants to say. These false starts make it difficult to follow the topic of his conversation. The scores from the NTLCE indicate that he is significantly below his age-matched peers on memory for commands, defining words, making judgments with syntax, and making a sentence. His scores are 1.5 to 2 standard deviations below the expected mean for his age. On the basis of the results of the NTLCE, it is clear that J. qualifies as a child with a language impairment. His scores on making judgments with syntax and making a sentence indicate that he has difficulty with language form, particularly with syntax. The analysis of his language sample also supports this. The next step in the process is to determine what treatment goals and objectives would be appropriate for J. The NTLCE has only indicated that J. needs some support in these areas, but it does not tell us specifically what kind of support J. needs. To write specific treatment goals for J. we will need to do additional assessment to determine appropriate goals and objectives for him.

Assessment to Determine Goals and Objectives

After we have established eligibility (determined that a child has a language impairment) goals and objectives must be written to address the individual learning profile of that child. As stated earlier, some information from the assessment to determine a diagnosis and eligibility will be useful as we write individualized goals and objectives; however, our assessment to determine a diagnosis and eligibility has some limitations for determining more specific goals and objectives:

- Most standardized tests provide a broad assessment of a range of language behaviors, not a detailed analysis of specifically what difficulties in language form, content, and use a child might have. In our hypothetical example, the NTLCE indicated that J. performed well below his age-matched peers in defining vocabulary words, indicating a deficit in language content. When we check the test protocol for defining words we note that J. defined eight words correctly but was unable to define the rest of the words before testing was discontinued. His ability to define eight words is certainly not enough information to write a goal or objectives for lexical acquisition.

- Because of the standardized administration procedures that must be followed when administering the test, a child's language abilities are assessed in an artificial environment. In our hypothetical example J.'s expressive language form was partially assessed by determining how well he was able to repeat a series of sentences presented by the examiner. This assessment procedure does not reflect how J. will use his expressive language in conversation to express his wants and needs with friends and adults. It also does not assess how J. communicates in the classroom in narrative and expository contexts to express what he knows to peers and his teachers.

- Because the test is administered in a structured environment, it is difficult to assess adequately language use or pragmatics to know how a child uses his language in realistic communicative contexts. The NTLCE provided no opportunities to determine how J. would request actions or objects, comment, refuse, state his position on an issue, or initiate, maintain, and terminate a conversation, for example. Thus, we know little of J.'s pragmatic abilities in naturalistic contexts from the NTCLE.

- Language comprehension and expression occur in naturalistic contexts with environmental supports to assist a child to communicate. These environmental supports include a predictable communicative context (playing with a friend, having a conversation with mom, describing something to a teacher) that the child has experienced before. Also included are visual supports and actions that help to define the context (toys, pictures, objects, other people interacting with these supports in meaningful ways). In the highly structured standardized test format all of these environmental supports are removed. In some situations there is no environmental support, simply the auditory message presented by the examiner (for example, in the sentence imitation subtest in the NTCLE, the student is asked to repeat a series of sentences read aloud by the examiner) or the support supplied from some two-dimensional pictures depicting an object, person or activity (the making of a sentence subtest of the NTLCE presents a series of pictures that a student will use to make different kinds of sentences).

- We have already mentioned that most of our standardized tests have a built-in cultural bias because they have been standardized on mainstream populations. Thus the results of these tests may lead to many false positives for children who are culturally and linguistically different from the children in the standardization sample.

- Many of the children seen by an SLP do not respond well to highly structured situations. Either these children will not be able to respond appropriately to complete the test or the results obtained do not represent a child's ability in more naturalistic contexts. Children with autism spectrum disorders (ASDs), for example, typically are not able to demonstrate their best abilities in these highly structured procedures. Many of our standardized language tests do not assess how a child will engage with a particular curriculum at a particular grade level, or what a child knows that will help her to meet the **educational benchmarks** for a particular grade. Many state departments of education define the specific skills and knowledge a student will gain at a particular grade level by establishing a series of benchmarks. **Table 4–2** presents some examples from the Michigan State Department of Education (2009) benchmarks in English and language arts for grade 4 students.

- The NTLCE does not assess how J. will use his language in the classroom to meet these benchmarks.

These are some of the reasons additional assessment is needed to determine individualized goals and objectives.

Criterion-Referenced, or Authentic, Assessments

The term **criterion-referenced assessment**, or **authentic assessment**, has sometimes been used to describe the informal or less standardized forms of assessments employed by SLPs (Robertson, 2007). Criterion-referenced implies that an examiner develops a set of necessary criteria to possess a particular language ability. Once the criteria are developed,

Table 4–2 Selected Michigan Benchmarks in English and Language Arts for Grade 4

English Language Arts Field Review
Participation and Supported Independence
Extended Grade-Level Content Expectations and Extended Benchmarks

Topic: Speaking, Speaking Conventions

Level of Independence Elementary School
(Full) (Linked to Grade 4)

ELA
Grade-Level Content Expectation v.12.05
S.CN.04.01
Use common grammatical structures correctly when speaking, including appositives, participial phrases, adjectives, adverbs, and prepositional phrases to express ideas in more complex sentences.

Classroom/State
S.CN.E.EG01
Make progress toward using grammatical structures, e.g., singular/plural nouns and simple conjunctions.

Classroom/State
S.CN.E.EG01
Make progress toward communicating accurately, e.g., speak in statements with simple conjunctions (*and, but, or*) rather than single words.

Topic: Speaking, Speaking Conventions (CN)

Level of Independence Elementary School
(Full) (Linked to Grade 4)

ELA
Grade-Level Content Expectation v.12.05
S.CN.04.02
Adjust their use of language to communicate effectively with a variety of audiences and for different purposes (e.g., community building, appreciation/ invitations, cross-curricular discussions), such as to inform or entertain diverse audiences.

Draft Supported Independence
Extended Grade-Level Content
Expectation/Extended Benchmark

(continued)

Table 4–2 (Continued)

Classroom/State
S.CN.E.EG02
Explore language to communicate with a variety of audiences and for different purposes, such as questions and answers with picture points.
Make progress toward maintaining effective body language for speaking; e.g., focus eyes toward audience and respect personal space.
Explore language to communicate with a variety of audiences and for different purposes, such as questions and answers with picture points.
Make progress toward communicating appropriately; e.g., listen while others are speaking; pause appropriately; use polite expressions such as *hello, good-bye, please*; respond appropriately to greetings.

English Language Arts Strand: Reading
Domain: Word Study (WS)

Level of Independence (Full) Elementary School, Middle School, High School
Assessable at:
(Classroom/State)
(Linked to Grade 4) (Linked to Grade 7)

ELA
Grade Level-Content Expectation v.12.05
R.WS.04.02
Use structural, syntactic, and semantic cues to automatically read frequently encountered words, decode unknown words, and decide meaning, including multiple meaning words (e.g., letter/sound, rhymes, base words, affixes, syllabication).

Classroom/State
R.WS.E.EG2
Use semantic and syntactic cues to recognize familiar words in context; e.g., understand familiar and functional words when they are paired with picture symbols, e.g., skull and crossbones paired with *poison*.

R.WS.E.EG02
Use semantic cues to recognize familiar words; e.g., select an object or a picture that is paired with a word.

Domain: Word Study (WS), Vocabulary

Level of Independence (Full) Elementary School, Middle School, High School
Assessable at:

Table 4–2 (Continued)

(Classroom/State)
(Linked to Grade 4) (Linked to Grade 7)

ELA
Grade-Level Content Expectation v.12.05
R.WS.04.07
In context, determine the meaning of words and phrases, including similes, metaphors, content vocabulary, and literary terms using strategies and resources, including context clues, semantic feature analysis, and a thesaurus.

R.WS.E.EG07
Show progress in recognizing words associated with familiar tasks.

Domain: Comprehension (CM)

Level of Independence (Full) Elementary School
Assessable at:
(Classroom/State)
(Linked to Grade 4)

ELA
Grade-Level Content Expectation v.12.05
R.CM.04.01
Connect personal knowledge, experiences, and understanding of the world to themes and perspectives in text through oral and written responses.

Classroom/State
R.CM.E.EG01
Connect words, pictures, personal knowledge, and experience to draw conclusions and make predictions about text.

R.CM.M.EG01
Connect words, pictures, personal knowledge

Classroom/State
R.CM.E.EG01
Use words, pictures, personal knowledge, and experience to draw conclusions about text.

Source: Courtesy of Michigan State Department of Education, 2009.

informal tasks are devised to elicit behaviors to assess each criterion. Authentic assessment is sometimes used to describe these procedures because they are thought to better reflect a child's ability as elicited in a more naturalistic and realistic context. Typically, these assessments are checklists of observations made of a child in an informal setting or protocols using naturalistic settings and materials administered in a more unstructured manner than standardized tests. These checklists and protocols may include classroom observations where appropriate, informal protocols developed originally as research instruments, or protocols developed by clinicians based on their clinical experience. Paul (2007) presents some examples of these informal protocols and checklists. She presents a checklist for assessing comprehension of the question words *what, where, who, whose, why* and *how many*. Informal checklists could also be constructed to assess comprehension of prepositions using favored objects. For J., we might develop some items that reflect the fourth-grade benchmarks listed in Table 4–2. For example, we could use objects or pictures to determine how he uses adjectives, adverbs, and prepositional phrases to describe what he sees. The speech and language assessment of J. included vocabulary items from his science, social studies, and language arts texts. This information will be used to write more specific goals and objectives regarding language content. When constructing these informal protocols, it is important to use the research in typical language acquisition to determine the appropriate ages for testing with a protocol and to determine the appropriate hierarchy of skills to be assessed.

There are particular concerns when informally assessing language comprehension because comprehension involves more than responding based on the words used in the assessment. Miller and Paul (1995) state that standardized tests fall short of full assessment of comprehension because they just assess the child's ability to decode "the literal meaning of isolated sentences" (p. 8). Comprehension is more than understanding the literal meaning of a phrase or sentence. It also includes extralinguistic knowledge often coded in the context, as well as the speaker's cues. In addition, comprehension in natural communicative contexts is embedded in levels of discourse. The discourse provides cues that can assist in comprehending a situation even though a child might not understand a particular phrase or sentence. Miller and Paul (1995) suggest that comprehension should be assessed in three tiers: (1) literal comprehension, (2) use of comprehension strategies, and (3) discourse features. Literal comprehension involves an assessment of a child's understanding of individual words and the associated grammatical structures in which those words are embedded.

The memory for commands subtest of the NTLCE is an example of literal comprehension. Assessing comprehension strategies involves observing how a child uses the context to respond to words or sentences that are too complex for him to understand, given his literal comprehension of the words and sentences. A classroom observation of J. might focus on observing carefully what J. is doing when the teacher gives a series of directions with commands. Is he employing any strategies to improve his comprehension? What visual or situational cues is he using to augment his understanding? Assessing discourse features determines how a child uses the structure of discourse to complement his understanding of language. For this level of comprehension, perhaps J.'s teacher needs to modify the language she uses in class when giving directions and instructions. She could modify her discourse to provide more clues and more opportunities for her class to hear the key words or concepts she wants them to understand. Readers are referred to Miller and Paul (1995) for a comprehensive set of procedures for assessing comprehension at these three levels.

Assessment of language use, or pragmatics, also needs to be determined in authentic informal assessments because language use is always embedded in a naturally occurring realistic context. Paul (2007) describes protocols that might be used to assess pragmatics informally:

- Craig (1991) assesses how children request, comment, make presuppositions about a listener, respond to a communicative partner, and adjust their speech style, and register to reflect different ages, different status, or different perspectives of listeners.
- Girolametto (1997) assesses a speaker's assertiveness and responsiveness. This profile is based on the work of Fey (1986).
- Prutting and Kirchner's Pragmatic Protocol (1983) assesses the variety of speech acts used by a child.
- Roth and Spekman (1984a, 1984b) suggested activities to assess comprehension and the use of communicative intentions, the understanding of presuppositions, and the ability to organize and engage in discourse.
- Creaghead's (1984) Peanut Butter Protocol worksheet assesses pragmatic abilities elicited in a structured snack setting.
- Ripich and Spinelli's (1985) Classroom Communication Checklist analyzes a child's communication in the classroom.
- Bedrosian's (1985) Discourse Skills Checklist analyzes topic initiation, maintenance, use of eye contact, turn-taking, politeness, and use of nonverbal behaviors.

For J., we could obtain some valuable information about his abilities to communicate in the classroom by using Creaghead's Peanut Butter Protocol, Ripich and Spinelli's Classroom Communication Checklist, and Bedrosian's Discourse Skills Checklist. These may be especially useful because of his teacher's concerns about his verbal abilities in class.

A common way to assess expressive language informally is to analyze a spontaneous language sample collected in conversation with a child. These procedures are intensive and time consuming. Paul (2007) suggests that we should not complete these analyses unless we have evidence in standardized testing or other observations that a child has impairments in language form in expressive language. Here are the general steps in using the sample to determine expressive language abilities:

- Record everything spoken in the conversation.
- Transcribe the recording including everything spoken by both participants.
- Select 50 to 100 fully intelligible **utterances** for further analysis.
- For children younger than 5 years, compute a **mean length of utterance** in morphemes (MLU).
- For school-aged children, analyze the sample for **T-unit** length in morphemes and narrative structure.
- Compare the MLU, T-unit to established normative data
- Determine the degree of development based on the normative data
- Analyze the sample for further aspects of language form. For younger children analyze the sample for Brown's (1973) **grammatical morphemes**. For older children, analyze for compound and complex sentence structure and narrative and discourse features (Miller, 1981; SALT, 2009)
- Analyze the sample for language content. Determine vocabulary diversity by computing a **type/token ratio (TTR)**, the **number of total words (NTW)** and the **number of different words (NDW)**.

The Systematic Analysis of Language Transcripts (SALT, 2009) is a computerized language sample analysis procedure many researchers and clinicians use to perform the analyses mentioned in this section after the sample is entered into the database. The Web site is http://www. saltsoftware.com/. The software is compatible with Windows XP and Vista.

Each step for manual analysis will now be discussed in detail.

The examiner records (video recording is a first choice; audio recording would be second) a spontaneous language sample. In this procedure, the examiner collects a sample by engaging in informal conversation with a child about the child's interests. Some researchers report that the examiner should have some rapport with the child for the sample to represent the child's best abilities (Bornstein, Haynes, Painter & Genevro, 2000), particularly for young preschool children (Owens, 2004). There are various issues to consider when collecting the sample:

- *Representativeness*: Is the sample a true picture of the child's typical conversation? A sample that contains many immediate repetitions of the adult model, that contains many fillers (*um, uh-huh, oh, yeah*), or that contains many rote or repetitive utterances, for instance, may not represent a child's true abilities (Miller, 1981).

- *How is the sample elicited?* There is no standardized way to elicit a sample. In general, the examiner should not to be too controlling in the interaction, should not use contrived procedures (e.g., sentence completion), but should elicit responses in an easy conversational manner. The examiner should attempt to follow the child's lead in the conversation (Cochrane, 1983). Miller (1981) provides some behaviors that would constitute good talking:
  - *Listen*: Follow the child's focus.
  - *Be patient*: Don't talk too much or try to initiate too often. Allow for periods of silence so that the child can initiate conversation.
  - *Follow the child's lead*: Provide a variety of choices to talk about. Allow the child to choose the topic, and then converse about her choices. Do not try to change the topic until the child signals in some way that she is ready to change.
  - *Do not ask dumb questions*: The conversation should center on what's happening in the moment. Do not waste time asking questions to which you both know the answer.
  - *Consider the child's perspective*: Be aware of how the child is viewing the situation. Choose materials and activities that match her cognitive and interest level. Respond to all attempts to communicate, and maintain appropriate affect.

- *What materials are used to elicit the sample?*
  - For preschool children, use favorite toys. Familiarity provides the knowledge so they know what to talk about.
  - For school-aged children, a more conversational style about their interests or school activities is likely to elicit more responses (Reed, 2005).

The examiner transcribes the entire recorded sample to obtain at least 50 utterances, although some reports suggest a sample of at least 100 utterances is more representative. There are a variety of methods for choosing utterances for further analysis. Regardless of the method, this is not a precise science. Owens (2004) presents the following guidelines for choosing utterances:

- A sentence constitutes an utterance.
- When there are not full sentences, use pauses, changes in intonation, and inhalations to mark utterance boundaries.
- Longer sentences containing a string of *ands* should be separated so that each utterance contains only one *and*.
- Longer compound and complex sentences with other conjunctions should stand as one utterance.
- Use the conversation in the transcription to determine utterance boundaries. The adult in the conversation may signal utterance boundaries by a response to the child.

For preschoolers, Miller (1981) suggests calculating the mean length of utterance (MLU) used by Brown (1973) in his longitudinal study of early language development. **Table 4–3** presents Miller's guidelines for calculating the MLU.

Appendix A presents a portion of a transcribed sample to illustrate how the MLU is computed. This is only a portion of the full sample. We should never compute an MLU on a sample this small.

Once the MLU is calculated, the obtained MLU is compared with normative data to determine the child's stage of development. If the MLU indicates some delay in development, then the sample should be analyzed for use of Brown's 14 grammatical morphemes. **Table 4–4** presents these morphemes.

Any morphemes determined to be missing or not used correctly in obligatory grammatical contexts should be further assessed using informal elicitation procedures to determine whether they are not used by the child or just did not occur in the sample obtained. Miller (1981) describes some procedures for eliciting particular morphemes not observed in the sample. Morphemes not used by the child become targets for intervention to increase the MLU to age-appropriate levels.

The MLU loses sensitivity as a marker of language growth as language gets more complex (Miller, 1981) because of increases in children's ability to use discourse features (Johnston, 2006; Paul, 2007). For older children, the T-unit is recommended to assess syntax in a conversational sample. The T-unit is one main clause with associated subordinating clauses and phrases. Clauses that use coordinating conjunctions *and* or

Table 4–3 Guidelines for Counting Morphemes

- All uninflected words equal one morpheme:
  (ex. *Dog, ball, juice, car, mommy*—each word = 1 morpheme)
- Words lacking semantic content are not counted
  (ex. *um, uh-huh, oops, oh*—each word = 0 morpheme)
- *Yeah, yes, no, hi, bye-bye*—each word = 1 morpheme
- Compound words equal one morpheme
  (ex. *Fire truck, choo-choo train, cluck-cluck, kitty cat*—each word = 1 morpheme)
- Irregular past tense verbs equal one morpheme
  (ex. *Saw, had, went, said, slept, did, ate, died*—each word = 1 morpheme)
- All auxiliary verbs equal one morpheme
  (ex. *Is* sleeping, *is* = 1 morpheme; *can* go, *can* = 1 morpheme; *will* ride, *will* = 1 morpheme, *gonna* go, *gonna* = 1 morpheme)
- All inflections count as one morpheme
  (ex. boy*s*, *s* = 1 morpheme; the girl*'s* dress, *'s* = 1 morpheme
  walk*ed*, *ed* = 1 morpheme; The boy see*s* the dog, *s* = 1 morpheme;
  he is walk*ing*, *ing* = 1 morpheme)

To Compute the Mean Length of Utterance:

1. Count the number of morphemes in each utterance.
2. Total the number of morphemes in the total sample.
3. Count the number of utterances included in the morpheme count.
4. Mean length of utterance = divide the total number of utterances by the total number of morphemes.

Source: Adapted from Miller, 1981.

but would be counted as separate T-units. We also look at the number of morphemes per T-unit. We would expect that the number of morphemes per T-unit will increase gradually through the school-age years and that greater increases in morphemes per T-unit would be seen in writing than in speaking (Nippold, 1998). Johnston (2006) recommends the mean length of utterance -2 (MLU2), a modification of the MLU, for older preschool children at later stages of MLU development. This method suggests removing imitative utterances from the sample, utterances that are single-word *yes/no* responses, and any utterances that are elliptical responses to a question. Elliptical responses are truncated utterances that occur in response to a question because the information is known in the context of the conversation and is supported by the discourse structure. For example:

Table 4–4 Brown's 14 Grammatical Morphemes

Morpheme	Example	Age of Mastery*
Present tense progressive -*ing*	He is sing**ing**.	19–28 months
In	He's **in** the house.	27–30 months
On	I'm **on** the table.	27–30 months
Regular plural -*s*	The girl**s** went home.	27–33 months
Irregular past	The mail **came** yesterday I **saw** that movie.	25–46 months
Possessive -*s*	The boy**'s** bicycle is gone.	26–40 months
Uncontractible copula (verb *to be* as main verb)	She **was** tired. **Is** it your car?	27–39 months
Articles *a, the*	**The** dog barked. I want **a** hot dog.	28–46 months
Regular past -*ed*	The bus stopp**ed** at the corner	26–48 months
Regular third person -*s*	He see**s** the fire truck.	26–46 months
Irregular third person	He **has** a new coat.	28–50 months
Uncontractible auxiliary (verb *to be* as auxiliary verb)	They **were** singing in the choir.	29–48 months
Contractible copula (verb *to be* as main verb)	She**'s** the one I saw yesterday He **is** the new president.	29–49 months
Contractible auxiliary (verb *to be* as auxiliary verb)	He**'s** running down the street.	30–50 months

Source: Adapted from Miller, 1981.

1. Adult: *Did you see Fluffy go outside?*
   Child: *No.*
   In this example, the child loses utterance length because there is
   no need to say, "I didn't see Fluffy go outside." The discourse
   supports the shared information between speaker and listener.

2. Adult: *Where did you put your sneakers?*
   Child: *Under my bed.*
   Again, in this example, the child loses utterance length because there is no need to say, "I put my sneakers under the bed." The discourse supports the shared information between speaker and listener.

Johnston (2001) compared the MLU2 procedure with the traditional MLU method in language samples from children 4 to 6 years, the highest ages for which the MLU procedure is recommended. She analyzed 24 samples from children with typical development and 23 from children diagnosed with language impairment. "For about one quarter of the children, MLU was altered by less than 10 percent. For about another quarter, it was altered by as much as 26 to 49 percent! Not surprisingly, samples in which the adult asked more questions were more affected by the alternate calculation method" (p. 116). She suggests that language sample comparisons used to determine progress (e.g., comparing a baseline sample and a sample after a period of treatment) should be elicited with similar discourse structures.

The sample is also analyzed for vocabulary diversity. Three methods appear in the literature: (1) the type/token ratio, (2) the number of different words, and (3) the number of total words.

- *Type/token ratio (TTR)*: The TTR is computed by counting the total number of words (the tokens) in a sample and dividing it by the total number of different words (the types). We would expect a ratio within the range of 0.45 to 0.55 to be typical if the sample is adequate (Templin, 1957).
- *Number of different words (NDW)*: The NDW is the count of the number of different words in a sample.
- *Number of total words*: The total number of words produced in a sample.

Watkins, Kelly, Harbers, and Hollis (1995) concluded that the NDW is better than the TTR as a measure of lexical diversity in samples of different utterance sizes. Klee (1992) states that the NDW and NTW are a better measure to use to determine language impairment because they actually discriminate between children with language impairments versus typically developing children. Normative data for NDW and NTW can be found in the SALT databases at http://www.saltsoftware.com/salt/downloads/referencedatabases.cfm.

Other informal measures have been suggested in addition to analyzing spontaneous language samples for assessing the language production of children. Seiger-Gardner (2009) discusses picture naming or confrontation naming, nonword and sentence repetition tasks, sentence completion tasks and elicited narratives as additional measures of language production. Picture-naming tasks require a child to identify an object or picture by retrieving the appropriate label from lexical storage and then saying the appropriate verbal label. This procedure is recommended to assess the word-finding abilities of children suspected of language content impairments. Children with word-finding difficulties have been found to have fewer words in their lexical storage and to be less efficient in retrieving information from storage (McGregor & Waxman, 1998; Newman & German, 2002; German & Newman, 2004). Nonword and sentence repetition tasks have been widely used in research to examine the abilities of children with language impairments. Nonword repetition tasks require a child to repeat a series of nonsense words presented verbally by an examiner. Studies support the use of the **nonword repetition** tasks as a culture-free means to assess phonological abilities and short-term memory. It has been used successfully to differentiate children with language impairments from children exhibiting typical development (Dollaghan & Campbell, 1998; Weismer, et al., 2000). The Children's Test of Nonword Repetition (CNRep), developed by Gathercole, Willis, Emslie, and Baddeley (1994), has been used widely in research. Many standardized tests of language ability use sentence repetition to assess the expressive abilities of children. In this task, the examiner verbally presents a series of sentences to a child and the child repeats the sentence as accurately as possible. Conti-Ramsden, Botting and Faragher (2001) and Botting and Conti-Ramsden (2003) found that a child's ability to repeat sentences accurately discriminates children with language impairment and children with ASD from children without language impairment. Sentence and story completion tasks are also used in some standardized tests. Sentence completion tasks, sometimes referred to as cloze procedures, require a child to complete a sentence that has missing words or grammatical elements presented verbally by an examiner. Elicited narratives are used widely to assess the discourse abilities of children. They can assess discourse features, such as sentence formulation, cohesive devices, narrative structures, and the general amount of language productivity (Seiger-Gardner, 2009).

The newest versions of the SALT analysis procedure include measures for analyzing language production in older children beyond the utterance level. The expository database has procedures for analyzing the **expository language** of middle and high school students. Expository language is used to explain how to do something. Teachers expect middle and high school students to communicate using expository language to demonstrate their understanding of concepts. The Edmonton Narrative Norms Instrument (ENNI) presents data on the narrative production of children aged 4 to 9 years. **Narratives** are descriptions of an event or a story. The conversation database presents samples of conversations of children aged 2;8 to 13;3 in which the children talk about topics such as classroom activities, holidays, family activities, and family pets. The Gillam Narrative Tasks Database presents narrative samples collected from 500 children aged 5;0 to 11 years. The normative samples of these databases are somewhat limited in terms of geographic distribution (students in Wisconsin; in Edmonton, Alberta, Canada; and in California), although the Gillam database reports on children from four geographic regions of the United States (Northeast, South, Midwest, and West). Nevertheless, these are valuable databases to assess the higher level language production of older school-aged children (SALT, 2009).

Dynamic Assessment

For older preschool and school-aged children, many researchers recommend using the principles of **dynamic assessment** to determine what kinds of supports a child needs to succeed in a given situation (Johnston, 2006; Merritt & Culatta, 1998). Most of the standardized tests currently used by SLPs assess language outside of the context of conversations and narratives and provide minimal support for a child to demonstrate learning. They also assume that testing a concept in one particular context determines what a child knows or does not know about that concept. Dynamic assessment is used to determine the learner's potential to acquire new knowledge. Vygotsky (1978) believed that learning is not a one-step process but, rather, a series of processes a learner engages in to acquire a concept. This series of processes is called the **zone of proximal development (ZPD)**. This zone is the learning edge for a child. Dynamic assessment in the classroom aims to assess this zone of acquisition by determining the following:

- What specific classroom tasks are difficult for the child?
- What language factors account for this difficulty?
- In what ways can the child's language be supported to make classroom learning more successful?
- What strategies can be taught to improve the child's language comprehension and production in the classroom?

- To what degree is the child successful in implementing strategies when the support is reduced? (Merritt & Culatta, 1998, pp. 106–107).

Dynamic assessment helps the SLP determine what kinds of supports a child needs to acquire a new concept or to be successful using the concept in meaningful contexts. For example:

- Does the repetition of a stimulus improve comprehension or performance?
- Does some form of visual support in terms of pictures or text improve comprehension or performance?
- Does allowing a different response (pointing versus verbalizing, one word versus a sentence, written versus spoken, written versus typed) from the child improve comprehension or performance?
- Does allowing more time to process and respond improve comprehension and performance?
- Does changing the complexity of language used in the task improve comprehension and performance?

When the clinician knows these things about a child's learning, the intervention can be better structured to assist concept acquisition and learning (Merritt & Culatta, 1998; Paul, 2007).

Special Considerations for Assessing Infants, Toddlers, and Young Preschoolers

The clinician engaged in assessing language and communication in young children needs to consider a particular set of issues:

- Family involvement and engagement
- The assessment setting
- Assessment materials
- The nature of the interaction
- Interpretation of responses
- Determining the prognosis

Family involvement and engagement is crucial during the assessment process. Because of developmental issues around attachment and separation we expect that the primary caregiver(s) will be intimately involved with the clinician as the assessment proceeds. The clinician needs to have particular skills in the areas of interviewing and communicating with families to ensure full engagement of the caregiver(s). Because the degree of involvement of the child is difficult to predict at these ages, the caregiver(s) may be the primary source of developmental information. It is important to elicit accurate case history information regarding pregnancy, birth, medical, cognitive, speech, language, and social issues. Engaging the family or caregiver(s) in the assessment process also helps to ensure engagement during intervention. Family and caregivers will be expected to be important intervention agents as treatment goals are implemented.

The assessment setting for young children is important to assure engagement. The setting should be well lit, comfortable, and have toys and materials that will engage a child's attention. The setting should be large enough to allow free movement if a child is ambulatory, but small enough to allow for control of movement and attention.

Assessment materials should be developmentally appropriate to elicit cognitive, social, and communication behaviors. To assess the range of abilities that might be exhibited by a child, a range of materials at different developmental levels should be available. Various toys and materials are also important so that the child will have multiple choices to engage attention. Families and caregivers may be asked to bring some of the child's favorite toys or games so that behaviors can be observed.

The nature of the interaction with caregivers is important for facilitating language and communication development. The clinician should structure the assessment session to obtain a valid assessment of the quality of the parent/caregiver and child interaction. Asking caregivers to interact with a child with a favorite toy or activity and observing him or her in play will usually provide a reliable observation. MacDonald's ECO Scales (MacDonald & Carroll, 1992) is a good instrument to assess the quality of the interaction observed. Likewise, the clinician needs to have particular skills to engage with the child appropriately. The clinician should also effectively use the principles of the ECO Scales to involve the child in communicative interaction.

Young children do not always respond as clearly as older children to assessment stimuli or to an interaction with a stranger. Therefore, the clinician may have to rely heavily on the caregiver to determine what kind of response the child made. A particular response may need to be elicited a number of times to determine the response's consistency. Young children may communicate in nonsymbolic or atypical ways (Owens, 2004). Caregivers are intimately acquainted with these behaviors and can help the clinician interpret what they are observing.

There are a number of parent report and observational instruments that may be used to determine the parent's estimation of how a child communicates at home. Perhaps the best validated instrument for toddlers is the MacArthur-Bates Communicative Development Inventories (CDI) (Fenson et al., 2006), also available in a Spanish version. The CDI have a version for children who are not yet combining words, the Words and Gestures Inventory, and another version for children who are producing sentences, the Words and Sentences Inventory. Both versions give families a standardized checklist of behaviors, words and gestures or words and sentences, to indicate which behaviors they see their child using at home. The checklist is then converted to a raw score that can be compared with normative data for typically developing children (8 to 18 months for the words and gestures, 16 to 30 months for the words and sentences). The Rossetti Infant-Toddler Scale (Rossetti, 2006) has a parent report form and an observational scale used by a clinician to assess interaction-attachment, pragmatics, play, gesture, language comprehension and language expression for children aged birth to 3 years. The Receptive-Expressive Emergent Language Test-3 (REEL-3) (Bzoch, League, & Brown, 2003) is an observational scale used by a clinician to assess language and communication development in children birth to 3 years. The test has a receptive language scale, an expressive language scale, and an inventory of vocabulary words.

Clinicians are required to provide families with a prognosis when the clinician has sufficient information to give one accurately. Determining the prognosis for young children may be problematic because it may be difficult to understand fully the course of development from the limited contact of an assessment, and because the course of development for young children over the coming years depends on a number of factors beyond the clinician's control. We do know that early and intensive intervention with full family support leads to better outcomes for young children (Paul, 2007).

Chapter Summary

There are a number of reasons children with language impairments need to be assessed, including to determine a diagnosis and eligibility and to determine goals and objectives. The assessment to establish eligibility can determine if the symptoms presented by a child characterize a language impairment and whether those symptoms are significant enough to warrant a diagnosis to establish eligibility for speech and language services. In this assessment, the SLP gathers all relevant background information about the child and family and then designs a series of procedures to assess the symptoms presented by the family and child. These procedures usually include some standardized tests, informal procedures to assess various aspects of language form, content, and use, and a spontaneous language sample. The standardized tests should be chosen carefully to ensure that they have appropriate validity and reliability and have an adequate normative sample. The SLP then analyzes the results of the evaluation to determine the nature and extent of the language impairment. If an impairment exists and an eligibility can be determined, then the SLP is charged with writing appropriate individualized goals and objectives for the child. The assessment to determine a diagnosis and eligibility usually does not provide enough information for the SLP to write adequate goals and objectives. This assessment samples a broad range of abilities in form, content, and use to determine how a child is functioning. Because this assessment is so broad, we typically do not have enough specific information about the child's abilities to write goals and objectives. Therefore, we then assess more specifically in selected areas, as determined by the assessment to establish eligibility, to write those goals and objectives. Criterion-referenced and authentic assessment procedures provide methods for assessing a child's abilities more specifically because they break language skills down into smaller developmental components, assess skills and abilities that may be more related to the curriculum, and allow the SLP to modify assessment procedures to see what modifications support the success of the child. There are special issues to address when assessing infants, toddlers, and preschoolers. These issues include involving and engaging the family, assessing the setting, assessing the materials, interacting, interpreting the responses, and determining the prognosis. The reliability and validity of the assessment of young children are improved when the clinician can modify assessment procedures to address these issues.

Terms from the Chapter

Authentic assessment *(56)*
Criterion-referenced assessment *(56)*
Dynamic assessment *(69)*
Educational benchmarks *(56)*

Eligibility *(46)*
Expository language *(68)*
Grammatical morphemes *(62)*
Mean *(48)*

Mean length of utterance *(62)*

Narratives *(69)*

Nonword repetition *(68)*

Normative sample *(48)*

Number of different words *(62)*

Number of total words *(62)*

Prognosis *(47)*

Reliability *(48)*

Scaled scores *(48)*

Standard deviation *(48)*

Standard error of measure *(51)*

T-unit *(62)*

Type/token ratio *(62)*

Utterance *(62)*

Validity *(52)*

Zone of proximal development *(69)*

References

Bedrosian, J. (1985). An approach to developing conversational competence. In D. Ripich and F. Spinelli (Eds.), *School discourse problems*. San Diego, CA: College Hill Press.

Bornstein, M., Haynes, O., Painter, K., & Genevro, J. (2000). Child language with mother and with stranger at home and in the laboratory: A methodological study. *Journal of Child Language, 27*, 407–420.

Botting, N., & Conti-Ramsden, G. (2003). Autism, primary pragmatic difficulties, and specific language impairment: Can we distinguish them using psycholinguistic markers? *Developmental Medicine & Child Neurology, 45*, 515–524.

Brown, R. (1973). *A first language: The early stages*. Cambridge, MA: Harvard University Press.

Bzoch, K. R., League, R., & Brown, V. L. (2003). *Receptive-expressive emergent language test* (REEL-3) (3rd ed.). Los Angeles, CA: Western Psychological Services.

Cochrane, R. (1983). Language and the atmosphere of delight. In H.Winitz. (Ed.), *Treating language disorders: For clinicians by clinicians*. Baltimore, MD: University Park Press.

Conti-Ramsden, G., Botting, N., & Faragher, B. (2001). Psycholinguistic markers for specific language impairment (SLI). *Journal of Child Psychology and Psychiatry, 42*, 741–748.

Craig, H. (1991). Pragmatic characteristics of the child with specific language impairment: An interactional perspective. In T. Gallagher (Ed.), *Pragmatics of language: Clinical practice issues* (pp. 89–100). San Diego, CA: Singular Press.

Creaghead, N. (1984). Strategies for evaluating and targeting pragmatic behaviors in young children. *Seminars in Speech, Language and Hearing, 5*, 241–252.

Dollaghan, C., & Campbell, T. F. (1998). Nonword repetition and child language impairment. *Journal of Speech, Language and Hearing Research, 41*, 1136–1146.

Fenson, L., Marchman, V., Thal, D., Dale, P., Reznick, S., & Bates, E. (2006). *MacArthur-Bates communicative development inventories (CDIs)* (2nd ed.). Baltimore, MD: Paul H. Brookes.

Fey, M. (1986). *Language intervention in young children.* San Diego, CA: College Hill Press.

Gathercole, S. E., Willis, C., Emslie, H., & Baddeley, A. D. (1994). The children's test of nonword repetition: A test of phonological working memory. *Memory, 2,* 103–127.

German, D. J., & Newman, R. S. (2004). The impact of lexical factors on children's word-finding errors. *Journal of Speech, Language, and Hearing Research, 47,* 624–636.

Girolametto, L. (1997). Development of a parent report measure for profiling the conversational skills of preschool children. *American Journal of Speech-Language Pathology, 6,* 33.

Johnston, J. (2001). An alternate MLU calculation: Magnitude and variablity of effects. *Journal of Speech, Language, and Hearing Research, 44,* 1362–1375.

Johnston, J. (2006). *Thinking about child language: Research to practice.* Eau Claire, WI: Thinking Publications.

Klee, T. (1992). Developmental and diagnostic characteristics of quantitative measures of children's language production. *Topics in Language Disorders, 12*(2), 28–41.

MacDonald, J., & Carroll, J. (1992). A social partnership model for assessing early communication development: An intervention model for preconversational children. *Language, Speech, and Hearing Services in Schools, 23,* 113–124.

McGregor, K. K., & Waxman, S. R. (1998). Object naming at multiple hierarchical levels: A comparison of preschoolers with and without word-finding deficits. *Journal of Child Language, 25,* 419–430.

Merritt, D. D., & Culatta, B. (1998). Language intervention in the classroom. San Diego, CA: Singular.

Michigan State Department of Education. (2009). Michigan education benchmarks. Retrieved August 23, 2009 from http://www.michigan.gov/mde/0,1607,7-140-28753---,00.html

Miller, J. F. (1981). *Assessing language production in children: Experimental procedures.* Baltimore, MD: University Park Press.

Miller, J. F., & Paul, R. (1995). *The clinical assessment of language comprehension.* Baltimore, MD: Paul H. Brookes.

Newman, R. S., & German, D. J. (2002). Effects of lexical factors on lexical access among typical language-learning children and children with word-finding difficulties. *Language and Speech, 45,* 285–317.

Nippold, M. (1998). *Later language development: The school-age and adolescent years.* Austin, TX: PRO-ED.

Owens, R. (2004). *Language disorders: A functional approach to assessment and intervention* (4th ed.). Boston, MA: Allyn and Bacon.

Paul, R. (2007). *Language disorders from infancy through adolescence: Assessment and intervention* (3rd ed.). Burlington, MA: Elsevier Science.

Prutting, C., & Kirchner, D. (1983). Applied pragmatics. In T. Gallagher (Ed.), *Pragmatics of language: Clinical practice issues.* San Diego, CA: Singular.

Reed, V. (2005). *An introduction to children with language disorders* (3rd ed.). Boston, MA: Allyn and Bacon.

Ripich, D. & Spinelli, F. (1985). (Eds.). *School discourse problems.* San Diego, CA: College Hill Press.

Robertson, S. (2007). Assessment of preschool and early school-age children with developmental language disorders. In A. Kamhi, J. Masterson, & K. Apel. (Eds.) *Clinical decision making in developmental language disorders* (pp. 39–54). Baltimore, MD: Paul H. Brookes.

Rossetti, L. (2006). *The Rossetti infant-toddler language scale.* East Moline, IL: LinguiSystems.

Roth, F., & Spekman, N. (1984a). Assessing the pragmatic abilities of children: Part 1. Organizational framework and assessment parameters. *Journal of Speech and Hearing Disorders, 49,* 2–11.

Roth, F., & Spekman, N. (1984b). Assessing the pragmatic abilities of children: Part 2. Guidelines, considerations and specific evaluation procedures. *Journal of Speech and Hearing Disorders, 49,* 12–17.

Seiger-Gardner, L. (2009). Language production approaches to child language disorders. In R. Schwartz (Ed.), *Handbook of child language disorders.* New York: Psychology Press.

Systematic analysis of language transcripts (SALT). (2009). Retrieved September 29, 2009 from http://www.saltsoftware.com

Templin, M. (1957). *Certain language skills in children: Their development and inter-relationships.* Minneapolis, MN: University of Minnesota Press.

Vygotsky, L. (1978). Mind in society: The development of higher psychological processes. Cambridge, MA: MIT Press.

Watkins, R., Kelly, D., Harbers, H., & Hollis, W. (1995). Measuring children's lexical diversity: Differentiating typical and impaired language learners. *Journal of Speech and Hearing Research, 38,* 476–489.

Weismer, S. E., Tomblin, J. B., Zhang, X., Buckwalter, P., Chynoweth, J. G., & Jones, M. (2000). Nonword repetition performance in school-age children with and without language impairment. *Journal of Speech, Language and Hearing Research, 43,* 865–878.

Appendix A Portion of a Transcribed Language Sample

Adult	Child	Morpheme Count
Setting: adult and a 3-year-old playing with a doll house.		
Oh, look at this.	1. What's this?	3
(pointing to the doorbell)		
	2. Can I press it?	4
Sure, let's see who comes	…	
to the door.	(unintelligible)*	
Who is it?	3. People	1
Yeah, there's people in there.	Yeah, people…	
	(partially intelligible)*	
Uh-huh.	4. What's this bed doing in here?	8
I think somebody sleeps there.	5. Not there.	2
	6. Right there.	2
Why are you putting it right here?	7. Cuz that's where the people sleep.	7
OK.	8. What's this?	3
I don't know, what do you think?	It's …	
	(partially intelligible)*	
Oh yes, I see.	9. Well, where's Matt?	4
Who's Matt, is he in there?	10. Yeah.	1
Where is he?	11. Let's open the garage.	4
OK, what do you see?	12. The car's in the house.	6
Number of morphemes = 45		
Number of utterances = 12	45/12 = 3.75	MLU = 3.75

*Note that partially intelligible or unintelligible utterances are not analyzed.

C H A P T E R   5

Intervention Goals

Bill Cupples

After reading this chapter you should be able to:

- Prioritize goals and objectives.
- Write goals and objectives in a particular format.
- Write goals and objectives in an appropriate sequence.
- Write goals and objectives in an appropriate hierarchy.
- Determine the appropriate criterion for a goal and an objective.
- Be able to baseline for an objective.
- Describe how the continuum of treatment affects goals and objectives.
- Describe various kinds of reinforcement.

Following the assessment to determine goals and objectives, the clinician engages in treatment planning to write the appropriate goals and objectives, to baseline those goals and objectives, to determine the best context for intervention, and to determine which intervention approach might be the most effective. As stated in Chapter 4, a thorough assessment using standardized tests, criterion-referenced, authentic, and dynamic assessments ensure that the clinician has the appropriate information to write goals and objectives.

Writing Goals and Objectives

Goals and **objectives** should be individualized for each particular child based on family input, the assessment data collected, and school input if age appropriate. Goals are generally considered long-term expectations of a child's performance and are typically included in the individualized family service plan (IFSP) of children younger than 3 years or the individualized education plan (IEP) for children older than 3 years and school age (Lignugaris-Kraft, Marchand-Martella & Martella, 2001; Paul, 2007). The long-term goals are further specified in terms of short-term objectives. These objectives are meaningful and intermediate steps we expect a child to achieve to meet the long-term goal. We write clear, concise, and specific goals and objectives because they keep our intervention clear and focused, provide a means for monitoring progress, help us to determine the outcomes of treatment and communicate to families, students, and other professionals what our plans are for a particular child (Lignugaris-Kraft et al., 2001).

Choosing Appropriate Goals and Objectives

Often a clinician must select a few behaviors for which goals and objectives might be written from many possible behaviors identified in the assessment (Hegde & Davis, 2005). Here are some suggestions for determining which of many targets might be chosen for goals and objectives:

- Prioritize targets that will have immediate impact on a person's communication skills.
- Prioritize targets that will be most useful in functional situations such as home and school.
- Prioritize targets that expand on existing behaviors or skills.
- Prioritize targets that are sensitive to cultural, social, and linguistic differences in the person's community.
- Choose targets that are priorities for the family.
- Prioritize targets that relate to educational **benchmarks** and the school curriculum and that are coordinated with classroom teachers (Michigan State Department of Education, 2009).

In addition to these considerations, targets should be chosen to represent a child's broad deficits. For instance, a child with deficits in language form, content, and use will need to have some goals and objectives written for each of those areas. Improving vocabulary (content) will give a child more words to use in sentences (form) and more in general to communicate in his social network and community (use). Owens (2004) emphasizes that language intervention should be placed in functional contexts and that language use, or pragmatics, is the determining or guiding component of the three. For example, we would target vocabulary (content) in contexts that are meaningful for a child (e.g., the classroom, the family, with peers); we would target sentence structure (form) in contexts in which a child would use the sentences (e.g., the classroom, the family, with peers).

The Structure of Goals and Objectives

The structure of a goal and its objectives will vary greatly depending on the context of treatment. Two ways of writing goals and objectives will be presented here. The Council for Exceptional Children presents a format for writing goals and objectives for an IEP (Lignugaris-Kraft, et al., 2001). The goal or objective has four components:

- The **condition**: the stimulus or stimulus situation that will be presented to a child
- The student name
- The clearly defined behavior: what specifically and behaviorally the student will do to demonstrate that he is addressing the goal and objective
- The performance criteria: how the behavior will be measured

An example of an objective written in this format would be as follows: given a picture of a volcano, Steven will verbally describe the processes that generate a volcano using at least five complete sentences and at least five vocabulary words from his science vocabulary as measured at least three times in 2 weeks in conversation with his clinician.

Roth and Worthington (2005) present the following components of a good goal or objective:

- The **do-statement**: what specifically the child will do to address the goal or objective
- The **stimulus condition**: the parameters of the stimulus (when the behavior will occur, what materials or cues will be used by the clinician, where or with whom the behavior will occur)
- The **criterion**: the expected level of performance

An example of an objective written in this format would be the following: Steven will use at least five words from his science vocabulary in at least five complete sentences in conversation with his clinician when presented with a picture of a volcano at least three times in the next 2 weeks.

Clinicians should choose the words carefully for the clearly defined behavior or the stimulus condition. Roth and Worthington (2005) discuss level 1 and level 2 verbs. Level 1 verbs include "point, label, repeat, match, name, tell, say, write, count, vocalize, ask" (p. 12). These are good verbs to use because it is clear what the child will do and what the clinician will count to keep data on the goal or objective. Level 2 verbs include "understand, think, learn, believe, improve, discover, know, appreciate, remember, apply, comprehend, feel" (p. 12). Although these are certainly skills we would like to see in students, these verbs are ambiguous for a goal or objective because it is not clear what the clinician will observe behaviorally from the child to demonstrate performance on the goal or objective. How does one observe and measure understanding, for instance? The child will have to do something more specific to demonstrate understanding.

As stated earlier, the objectives for a goal are the steps or sequence of learning through which we expect a child to progress to reach the goal. These objectives are usually arranged in a sequence or in a **hierarchy**. An example of objectives that might be written in a sequence is objectives written for a child to be able to dress himself. Obviously, underwear would go on first and then the shirt, the pants, the socks, and the shoes. In speech and language an example of a sequence would be objectives that would be written as a social script for an adolescent. For example, what would you do first after entering a room of your peers, what would you do second, what would you do third, and so forth. Most frequently for children with language impairments, objectives are written in hierarchies. These may be developmental hierarchies such as the following:

- Produces vocabulary of single words, mostly nouns
- Produces two-word utterances with nouns, verbs, and pivots
- Produces two-word utterances *with here, there, that, want, wanna, up, down, I, you* and with the grammatical morphemes plural *–s* and progressive *-ing*
- Produces three or more word utterances with more grammatical morphemes (Johnston, 2006)

There are hierarchies of complexity of verbal response:

- In single, monosyllabic words
- In single, multisyllabic words
- In phrases
- In sentences
- In conversation

There are hierarchies of stimulus type:

- Direct physical manipulation
- Concrete symbols

- o Objects
- o Photographs, colored pictures
- o Black-and-white line drawings

- Abstract symbols
  - o Oral language
  - o Written language (Roth & Worthington, 2005)

There are also hierarchies based on using educational benchmarks for a given grade. **Table 5–1** is a hierarchy for **phonemic awareness** from the first-grade Michigan educational benchmarks.

Determining the expected criterion for a goal or objective is not always clear. Ultimately, a child should be expected to use a given behavior at a high level of proficiency. Research in applied behavioral analysis has suggested that a criterion of 80 percent would be considered a mastery level. The Feuerstein method (2009) suggests that mastery is not what we want; he suggests that learning at a 50 to 60 percent level keeps a child from being too prompt or stimulus dependent (R. Liepack, personal communication, May 22, 2009).

Clinicians also have to decide whether criterion will be measured in percentage correct or in frequencies. Percentage criteria are usually good for objectives written for activities that will present stimuli in **discrete trials**. Discrete trials occur when a clinician presents a given stimulus (e.g., a picture) and requests a given response (e.g., the client labels the picture with the appropriate name or produces the label with a given phoneme) (Hegde & Davis, 2005). In this situation the clinician knows how many stimuli will be presented because she knows how many pictures she will present or how many specific productions will be requested. For example, if we know that we will present 20 pictures to a child we know that there will be 20 opportunities for the child to produce the target. A percentage is easy to compute in a therapy task like this (e.g., the client produces 16 of 20 responses correctly; the percentage correct is 80 percent). Discrete trials are not naturalistic, however. Discrete trials are clinician directed and present stimuli in a highly structured situation (Prizant & Wetherby, 1998). Children do not typically learn in these highly structured situations but, rather, learn in naturalistic contexts like play or in school, contexts that are not structured in discrete trials. In these contexts, we cannot predict in advance how many times a given stimulus will be presented or how many opportunities a child will have to exhibit a particular behavior. When this information is lacking, it is difficult to compute a percentage. The following example presents a more naturalistic situation.

Table 5–1 Phonemic Awareness

Students will...

Demonstrate phonemic awareness by the wide range of sound manipulation competencies, including sound blending and deletion.

Recognize that words are composed of sounds blended together and carry meaning.

Phonics
Students will...

Understand the alphabetic principle, that sounds in words are expressed by the letters of the alphabet.

Use structural cues to recognize one-syllable words, blends, and consonant digraphs, including letter-sound, onset and rhymes, whole-word chunks, word families, digraphs *th, ch, sh.*

Word Recognition
Students will...

Automatically recognize frequently encountered words in and out of context with the number of words that can be read fluently increasing steadily across the school year.

Make progress in automatically recognizing the 220 Dolch basic sight words and 95 common nouns for mastery in third grade.

Use strategies to identify unknown words and construct meaning by using initial letters/sounds (phonics), patterns of language (syntactic), picture clues (semantic), and applying context clues to select between alternative meanings.

Use syntactic and semantic cues, including picture clues, word chunks, and the structure of book language to determine the meaning of words in grade-appropriate texts.

Know the meanings of words encountered frequently in grade-level reading and oral language contexts.

Source: Adapted from Michigan State Department of Education, 2009.

A Case Study

J.'s clinician has been working with him in therapy to increase his use of questions to solicit information. He has succeeded in the structured therapy situation to use questions to gather more information. His clinician now wants to work on generalizing this behavior to his classroom. She works in the classroom with him to prompt him to ask questions during a science class when he does not understand directions or a given concept.

In this situation, the clinician cannot predict how many opportunities the teacher will provide for J. to ask questions, how many questions J. will ask, or whether another student will ask a question that clarifies the information for J. Frequency of response would be an easier criterion to use to measure progress toward the objective since we do not know how many trials or opportunities J. will have to use questions. In general, in more naturalistic contexts the clinician will write an objective using frequency as the criterion.

Baselines for Goals and Objectives

Before beginning work on an objective the clinician needs to determine the client's abilities for that particular target. **Baselines** are measurements of a behavior in the absence of treatment (Hegde & Davis, 2005). It is important to determine baseline functioning to know where we are starting with a particular behavior and to track progress on that behavior as we implement treatment. Accurate baselines mean that the objective is appropriate (i.e., the client cannot perform the targeted behavior) and that we have a clear idea of where we are starting to determine the outcome of treatment for that particular set of objectives and the associated goal. Baseline tasks should be structured to meet the following criteria:

- Baseline only those behaviors that will be treated immediately in order to have the most recent data on the client's abilities.
- Tasks used to elicit the behavior should have clear and concise instructions so that the client knows precisely what is expected.
- The baseline task should provide enough opportunities to elicit the desired behavior in the appropriate context.
- To be reliable, elicit enough responses in the appropriate context to have a clear idea of the child's abilities.
- Record the client's responses accurately and write objective statements to describe the client's performance.
- Objective statements should include percentage or frequency counts for a given behavior.

How to Baseline a Given Behavior

A baseline is a mini-assessment of a particular behavior. The following decisions need to be made to design a baseline procedure:

- Determine the number of times a given behavior should be elicited
- Choose the activity or material to elicit the behavior
- Determine how the behavior will be measured
- Determine how the behavior will be elicited

Many of the informal procedures discussed in Chapter 4 could be adapted to use as a baseline. A baseline for the production of grammatical morphemes might include the following:

- Elicit the plural –s at least 20 times.
- Pictures of single objects and pictures of two or more of the same objects.
- A checklist of the 20 trials is constructed; responses will be recorded on the checklist.
- Use questions to elicit responses when each picture is presented (*What is this? What are these?*).

A baseline for a child's use of narrative structures might include the following:

- Elicit two or three narratives.
- Have a conversation with a child.
- Ask the child to tell you about a time she was hurt, to explain how to order food in a restaurant, and to tell a story using a wordless picture book (Paul, 2007).
- Assess the transcript for the level of narrative development (additive chain, temporal chain, causal chain, multiple causal chain) (Lahey, 1988).
- Observational scales might also be used to baseline a behavior. Ripich and Spinelli's (1985) Classroom Communication Checklist analyzes a child's communication in the classroom. The clinician could observe a child in a particular activity in the classroom for about 30 minutes and complete the checklist during the observation.

Baselines for Early Intervention

In general, the baselines for early intervention are obtained in naturalistic contexts in interaction with caregivers and adults (Paul, 2007). These naturalistic contexts include daily routines, such as dressing, playing, and interacting with peers. Baselines obtained in these environments ensure that we have an authentic assessment of behavior because we have assessed behaviors in familiar routines and in situations where a child will be highly motivated to communicate. The following are some typical behaviors we might want to baseline in early intervention for infants and toddlers:

• Quality of the interaction between caregiver and child
• Nonverbal versus verbal communication
• Use of gestures to communicate
• Use of intentional communication
• Understanding of developmentally appropriate vocabulary
• The number of words in the expressive vocabulary
• The pragmatic purpose of communication (give, request actions, request objects, show, refuse, deny, comment)
• Comprehension of developmentally appropriate commands or instructions
• Semantic meanings and length of utterances produced (Johnston, 2006; Owens, 2004)

Baselines for Preschool Intervention

In preschool, intervention baselines are usually obtained in structured play situations in interaction with adults and peers. Because of emergent literacy in older preschoolers, we could expect that pictures or books might be used also to elicit certain targets. Here are some examples of behaviors that might be baselined:

• Interaction between caregiver and child
• Nonverbal versus verbal communication
• Understanding of developmentally appropriate vocabulary
• The number of words in the expressive vocabulary
• The pragmatic purpose of communication (give, request actions, request objects, request clarification, show, refuse, protest, comment, answer, acknowledge, hypothesize, predict)
• Comprehension of developmentally appropriate commands or instructions
• Use of developmentally appropriate grammatical forms
• Conversational abilities (topic selection, introduction and maintenance, turn-taking, adjacency, and contingency of responses)
• Use of narratives to describe events and activities
• Phonological awareness and word knowledge (Owens, 2004; Paul, 2007).

Baselines for School-Aged Intervention

School-aged baselines are usually obtained in interaction with the clinician, with peers, and in classrooms. Baselines will include assessment of spoken and written language. Here are some examples of behaviors that might be assessed for baselines:

- Phonological awareness
- Understanding of developmentally appropriate vocabulary
- The number of words in the expressive vocabulary
- The pragmatic purpose of communication (give, request actions, request objects, request clarification, refuse, protest, comment, answer, acknowledge, hypothesize, predict)
- Conversational abilities (topic selection, initiation and maintenance, turn-taking, adjacency, and contingency of responses)
- Politeness (understanding and using indirect requests and commands, use of polite terms)
- Understanding and using narratives to describe events and activities in speaking and in writing
- Understanding and using fictional narratives in speaking and writing
- Understanding and using expository language in speaking and writing
- Understanding and using humor (irony, violations of presuppositions, sarcasm)
- Understanding and using metaphorical language (idioms, similes, and metaphors)
- Understanding and using complex syntax (additive chains, temporal chains, causal chains)
- Understanding and using concepts in educational benchmarks for an expected grade level (Merritt & Cullatta, 1998; Owens, 2004; Paul, 2007).

A clinician who obtains accurate baseline measures has a clear picture of a child's current abilities and has a clear idea of where to begin intervention.

Goals and Objectives and the Continuum of Treatment

The form of goals and objectives and the data collection for goals and objectives will vary depending on the type of intervention employed by the clinician. As discussed in Chapter 6, the form of intervention may vary depending on where a particular approach falls on the continuum of treatment. At one end of the continuum are **clinician-directed (CD)** approaches such as discrete trials. At the other end of the continuum are approaches that are **child centered (CC)** (Fey, 1986). Prizant and Wetherby (1998) describe the continuum from discrete trials (DT) at one end to **developmental-social-pragmatic (DSP)** approaches at the other end.

Those using clinician-directed approaches often write goals and objectives in the format discussed earlier in this chapter. Usually, the criteria in these goals and objectives can be measured using percentage correct because clinician-directed approaches often involve using discrete trials. As we move further along the continuum to CC or DSP approaches, it becomes more difficult to measure a child's performance in percentages because we move further away from discrete trial approaches. Frequency counts of behavior are more appropriate for these types of intervention.

Variations in the Stimulus Condition

The stimulus condition of goals and objectives is also different, depending where an intervention approach falls on the continuum. In CD interventions the clinician carefully selects a set of stimuli to elicit a particular response from a child. This careful stimulus selection means that the stimulus condition can be stated succinctly and clearly. As we use approaches further along the continuum to CC or DSP approaches, we find that the stimuli are more varied and the stimulus context is more complex. For example, in a CC approach, the child chooses the materials and activities for the intervention session (Prizant & Wetherby, 1998); the clinician cannot predict in advance which of the various stimuli the child will choose. Thus, the stimulus condition will be more general (e.g., in structured play, during meals, in conversation with a peer).

Variations in the Recipient of Goals and Objectives

In CD approaches, goals and objectives are written for the child with the language impairment. In CC or DSP approaches, goals and objectives may be written for adults in the situation to support the discourse features of a conversation. For example, caregivers may have goals written to improve their ability to use utterances closer to the developmental level of their child. They may have goals written to use various types of questions to elicit more responses from their child. They may have goals written to modify their directiveness or responsiveness with their child.

Variations in the Stimulus Context

The continuum of treatment may also determine the stimulus context. In DT or CD approaches, the clinician usually carefully controls the context. Most often, the context is a clinical context or a carefully constructed context in the child's home. As stated earlier, the clinician carefully selects and presents stimuli to elicit the desired behavior. In CC or DSP approaches, the more naturalistic context means that there are more stimuli and the context is richer. A preschool classroom, a child's home, or an elementary classroom is a rich context, full of stimuli and environmental supports to elicit a given behavior.

Variations in Reinforcement

The kind and types of reinforcement will vary depending on the type of intervention employed. CD and DT approaches usually employ specific reinforcement schedules to ensure that the target behavior is acquired. For instance, initially every correct response is reinforced (continuous schedule reinforcement). As the child demonstrates success with achieving the target the reinforcement schedule is modified to an intermittent reinforcement schedule. Intermittent reinforcement can be given after a set number of correct responses (fixed ratio schedule), after an average number of correct responses (variable ratio schedule), after a specified time period (fixed interval schedule) or after a varying time period (variable interval schedule) (Hegde & Davis, 2005). CD and DT approaches will also use token reinforcement to increase target behaviors. Token reinforcement may include presenting food, favorite toys, or access to favorite activities when a target behavior occurs. In CC or DSP approaches, because the child directs the session and chooses the toys or activities, the reinforcement in the session is intrinsic. In other words, because the child is interested in the activity, engagement in the activity provides the pleasurable experience that motivates the child to continue the activity. In addition, the persons interacting with the child in the activity use social reinforcement when desired behaviors occur. Social reinforcement includes positive affect, such gestures as high-five, and using words like super, great job, awesome, and that's it.

Johnston (2006) states that the use of the word *reinforcement* in treatment sessions is inappropriate. Adults reinforce a desired behavior, so the motivation to respond is external to the child. She believes that, if we structure intervention with toys, materials, activities, and contexts that reflect a child's interests, motivation to participate in the activity will mitigate the need for externally applied reinforcement. Koegel and Koegel (2006) describe motivation as one of the pivotal elements in their treatment program. They maintain that we should design programs on the basis of children's natural motivations. If we base our intervention programs on children's choices for what motivates them, then we are more likely to develop functional skills that will **generalize** automatically to other contexts.

Chapter Summary

Goals and objectives are written to provide individualized, measurable steps in a treatment program. Goals are generally considered to be more long-term, generalized sets of expectations, while objectives are the specific sets of expectations we have for a child during treatment. There are many ways to write goals and objectives. This chapter presents two ways to structure goals and objectives. First, objectives are written in hierarchies, with clinicians starting with simpler skills and abilities in the hierarchy that match a child's current level of performance. The current level of performance is determined by obtaining a baseline, a measure of a given skill or ability before initiating treatment. Second, goals and objectives vary depending on the type of treatment approach used by a clinician. Treatment approaches in speech and language pathology vary along a continuum. The continuum is defined by clinician-directed, highly structured approaches on one end to child-centered, child-directed, more flexible approaches at the other end. Goals and objectives change in terms of the stimulus condition, the recipient of the goal or objective, the stimulus context, and variations in reinforcement as we move along the continuum of treatment.

Terms from the Chapter

Baseline *(85)*

Benchmark *(80)*

Child centered *(89)*

Clinician-directed *(89)*

Condition *(81)*

Criterion *(81)*

Developmental-social-pragmatic *(89)*

Discrete trials *(83)*

Do-statement *(81)*

Generalization *(91)*

Goals *(79)*

Hierarchy *(82)*

Objectives *(79)*

Phonemic awareness *(83)*

Stimulus condition *(81)*

References

Feuerstein, R. (2007). A mediational approach to teaching and learning. Retrieved from http://www.feuersteintraining.co.uk/mediational.htm

Fey, M. E. (1986). *Language intervention with young children*. San Diego, CA: College Hill Press.

Hegde, M. N., & Davis, D. (2005). *Clinical methods and practicum in speech-language pathology* (4th ed.). Florence, KY: Cengage Learning.

Johnston, J. (2006). *Thinking about child language: Research to practice*. Eau Claire, WI: Thinking Publications.

Koegel, R., & Koegel, L. (2006). *Pivotal response treatments for autism: Communication, social, and academic development*. Baltimore, MD: Paul H. Brookes.

Lahey, M. (1988). *Language disorders and language development*. New York, NY: Macmillan Publishing.

Lignugaris-Kraft, B., Marchand-Martella, N., & Martella, R. (2001). Writing better goals and short-term objectives or benchmarks. *Teaching Exceptional Children, 34*, 52–58.

Merrit, D. D., & Cullatta, B. (1998). *Language intervention in the classroom*. San Diego, CA: Singular Publishing Group.

Michigan State Department of Education. (2009). Michigan first grade english and language arts grade level content expectations. Retrieved from http://www.michigan.gov/mde/0,1607,7-140-28753_33232---,00.html

Owens, R. (2004). *Language disorders: A functional approach to assessment and intervention* (4th ed). Boston, MA: Allyn and Bacon.

Paul, R. (2007). *Language disorders from infancy through adolescence: Assessment and intervention* (3rd ed.) Burlington, MA: Elsevier Science.

Prizant, B., & Wetherby, A. M. (1998). Understanding the continuum of discrete-trial traditional behavioral to social-pragmatic developmental approaches in communication enhancement for young children with autism/PDD. *Seminars in Speech and Language, 19*, 329–353.

Ripich, D., & Spinelli, F. (Eds.). (1985). *School discourse problems*. San Diego, CA: College Hill Press.

Roth, F., & Worthington, C. (2005). *Treatment resource manual for speech-language pathology*. Clifton Park, NY: Thomson Delmar Learning.

CHAPTER 6

Approaches to Intervention

Ronald B. Hoodin

Chapter Objectives

After reading this chapter, you should be able to:

- Describe treatment as a form of hypothesis testing.
- Discuss the clinician's influence over the linguistic environment of treatment.
- Discuss the clinician's control over the nonlinguistic stimuli brought to treatment.
- Discuss the continuum of naturalness that serves as a basis for describing a broad range of eclectic treatments.
- Discuss the clinician-directed approaches to treatment.
- Discuss the child-centered approaches to treatment.
- Discuss the hybrid approaches to treatment.
- Discuss the three levels of intervention: acquisition, maintenance, and generalization.

Treatment or intervention in the field of childhood language disorders is an important topic that deserves to be discussed objectively. Treatment consists of variables that can be measured and manipulated (Hegde, 1994). The emphasis is on two kinds of variables: independent and dependent variables. **Independent variables** are the causes or treatments, whereas **dependent variables** are the effects or responses. Conceived in this manner, implementing treatment is engaging in a scientific methodology called **hypothesis testing**. The implicit hypothesis is that the treatment will be effective. This view of treatment casts the clinician in the role of clinician–researcher.

To continue this reasoning, during intervention, the clinician provides a particular set of stimulus conditions that reflect the selected treatment approach. The child provides the responses that, according to the implicit hypothesis, are modified by the treatment. These stimulus conditions are described later within the context of each of the treatment approaches.

Beyond selecting a treatment procedure, clinicians influence both the linguistic environment of intervention by controlling their own speech and the nonlinguistic context of intervention by selecting materials to be used. Sheng, McGregor, and Xu (2003) described variations in clinicians' speech to accommodate the child's age and diagnostic status. These variations, which they called **therapeutic register**, included reducing rate, reducing sentence complexity, increasing repetitions, increasing pause time, and using exaggerated prosody with young or linguistically impaired children. Paul (2007) discussed the nonlinguistic stimuli that clinicians bring to intervention, which often include pictures, toys, and real objects. She noted that clinicians prefer pictures because they are easy to access and handle. However, pictures may not always be the best choice. For example, a picture of a ball will not roll. Therefore, pictures cannot fully represent objects. The implication is that clinicians should have a variety of nonlinguistic stimuli available rather than relying solely on pictures.

A Continuum of Naturalness

Fey (1986) proposed a **continuum of naturalness** for describing a broad range of eclectic treatment approaches. He identified three factors that determine treatment naturalness, including (1) the particular treatment activity as well as (2) the physical and (3) the social context of treatment. At the low end of the continuum are highly structured, artificial, and drill-like treatment activities that take place in unfamiliar surroundings, such as at a clinic, and are administered by a stranger, such as a clinician. At the high end of the continuum are loosely structured treatment activities, such as everyday activities that take place in familiar surroundings, like at the child's home, and are carried out by family members. Other treatment approaches fall along the continuum at intermediate positions, as they borrow elements from each end. The continuum of naturalness is not a formal scale (Hepting & Goldstein, 1996). It is simply a convenient mechanism for describing approaches to treatment. Clinicians should feel free to select procedures from any place along the continuum, to combine procedures into packages, and to move along the continuum as their judgment indicates.

Clinician-Directed Approaches

At the low end of the continuum of naturalness are the **clinician-directed (CD) approaches**. In using the CD approaches, the clinician predetermines the goals, activities, correct responses, and criteria set for mastery. Various training procedures to improve the child's language skills are used in the CD approaches. These procedures typically occur within **discrete trials**, which are structured opportunities for training. The term *discrete* is used because a pause is inserted to distinguish one opportunity from the next. The clinician may instruct the child concerning the **target response**—the response being taught. The clinician also provides **training stimuli** for eliciting target responses. Training stimuli, such as pictures, are carefully planned and controlled. It is common for clinicians to use models. A **model** is a correct production of the target response the child will imitate. When the target response is not forthcoming, the clinician may provide a prompt. **Prompts** are requests, hints, or cues designed to help elicit the target response. Prompts and models are often **faded**, that is, gradually reduced as the child begins to acquire the target form. When the child produces the target response, the clinician may provide reinforcement.

Reinforcement is a type of consequence that increases the frequency of the behavior. Reinforcement is referred to as **extrinsic reinforcement** when candy, stickers, and praise are used, because these reinforcements do not occur during natural communication. Conversely, **intrinsic reinforcement** naturally arises in the communicative context. For example, if a young child requests some juice and gets it, then the requesting behavior has been intrinsically reinforced because it occurs naturally. The notions of feedback and reinforcement are related because both are consequences. However, **feedback** is used to provide information regarding the correctness of the child's response. **Shaping**, another training procedure, refers to gradually modifying a response until the target response is elicited. It is usually employed with complex target responses. To use shaping, an incomplete or otherwise deficient form of the target response is initially reinforced until it is consistently elicited. Then, the response is only reinforced when it corresponds more closely to the target response. This incremental strategy may continue for several steps until the target response is actually elicited. Examples of the CD approach can be seen in Chapter 10: exemplars 1, 4, 8, 10, and 20.

To minimize boredom, which may accompany the drill-like quality associated with the CD approaches, some clinicians introduce an additional motivator into the structure of the activity (Paul, 2007). An example would be a game format in which, with the roll of the dice, the child moves his token on a game board and drama ensues. At strategic moments in the game, the child is required to use the target response or his token becomes imperiled.

In general, the CD approaches have been used successfully with a heterogeneous group of children. However, CD approaches are not for everyone. Some children do not adapt well to the structure associated with the CD approaches (Fey, 1986; Paul, 2007). These include children who are obstinate, unassertive, or immature. Such children may respond better to more naturalistic approaches.

The CD approaches may also be applied to teaching advanced language forms in the school years and beyond. During the school years, most children acquire **metalinguistic ability**, the ability to consciously reflect on language. Metalinguistic skills promote language acquisition, especially in advanced forms, including figurative language (Wallach & Miller, 1988). School-aged children are expected to learn **figurative language**, including idioms, similes, metaphors, and proverbs, that are in common usage. However, language-impaired children are behind in this (Wallach & Miller, 1988). Therefore, figurative language represents an important treatment target for school-aged children.

Teaching students to explain metaphors serves as an example of using metalinguistic skills to train figurative language in the context of the CD approaches. A **metaphor** describes one referent in terms of another, for example, "My daughter is a jewel." To understand this sentence, the listener rejects the literal message, which is absurd, yet marks the presence of the metaphor and simultaneously provides clues to the intended message. That is, a jewel is precious, so the underlying message is that my daughter is precious. The clinician first increases the student's metalinguistic awareness of the nature of metaphors and then applies behavioral procedures to teach the student to explain the metaphor.

To increase metalinguistic awareness of metaphors, Wallach and Miller (1988) suggest explaining the nature of metaphors by using multiple-choice fill-ins, riddles, and explicit sentences to illustrate the similarity between two referents. An example of a fill-in is, "The speedboat _____ " where A. "traveled fast," is literal and B, "was a rocket" is metaphorical. An example of a riddle is, "What spins like a top but does so on the ice?" The answer is a figure skater. Finally, an example of a sentence that makes the similarities between two referents explicit is, "A giraffe is tall like a flagpole." As shown, fill-ins, riddles, and explicit sentences highlight the similarity between two referents as a means of developing metalinguistc awareness of the nature of metaphors.

After gaining a sense of the nature of metaphors, the student is ready to learn to identify and explain individual metaphors. The clinician begins by using a series of metaphors in a monologue. Every time a metaphor is used the student is required to identify it. Then, the student is asked to explain it. During these attempts, the clinician uses prompts to guide the student. As the student acquires the target skill, the prompts are faded.

Child-Centered Approaches

At the high end of the continuum of naturalness are the **child-centered (CC) approaches**. According to Fey (1986), the basic objective of the CC approaches is to place the child in a highly accepting, responsive environment that motivates the child to communicate spontaneously. This environment is generally arranged as **facilitative play**. That is, the clinician may be trying to entice the child into communicating, but from the child's perspective, the activity is just play. The general stimulation procedure is used in the context of facilitative play.

General Stimulation

The clinician arranges an inviting environment for the child. Choices or alternative play materials are presented. The clinician sits on the floor adjacent to the child and engages in parallel play with the child using the materials that the child selected. Both the child and the clinician play with the same toys, such as toy cars. Then, the clinician begins the **general stimulation** procedure. That is, the clinician starts talking about what he or she is doing so that the child can see a close match between the clinician's words and actions. For example, "I am making the car go. The car is going. See the car go." The child will likely attend to the clinician because after all, the child selected the materials, suggesting that the activity is interesting. Furthermore, the clinician speaks in an animated fashion, which attracts the child's notice. By engaging in general stimulation, the clinician provides a model for imitation although no demands are made on the child. Shaping and prompting are not used. Instead, the clinician follows the child's lead and responds. After providing the model, the clinician waits expectantly for the child to respond. When the child responds, the clinician interprets the child's behavior as meaningful and communicative, even if it is not. These activities are intrinsically rewarding, so the clinician does not provide extrinsic reinforcement. According to Hubbell (1981), intrinsic reinforcement places behavior modification in the context of communication, which is natural.

Conversely, extrinsic reinforcement places communication in the context of behavior modification, which is contrived. Therefore, intrinsic reinforcement is preferred in this approach. When the child responds verbally, the clinician imitates the child. Even though the child is not required to imitate, it is likely that the child will imitate the imitation. When the child imitates, this may encourage a turn-taking-type dialogue. That is, the child initiates, the adult responds, and then it is the child's turn again and so on. This encourages an ongoing, turn-taking quality, which characterizes natural conversations. Children often imitate adult models, so taken together, these techniques maximize the chance that the child will make a spontaneous utterance. Another example of the CC approach can be seen in exemplar 22 in Chapter 10.

The CC approaches are not for every child (Fey, 1986; Paul, 2007). If the child is an assertive and responsive communicator but exhibits deficiencies in specific linguistic forms, then other approaches would be preferable. The CC approaches are not capable of addressing specific language goals. However, if the child is passive or refuses to participate in CD approaches, then the child is a good candidate for the CC approaches. Because no demands are made on the child, the child does not use his or her energies to resist. Instead, the child may respond in a more natural fashion. Therefore, the CC approaches represent a good starting point for such a child. When the child reaches the level of regularly contributing to conversations, then the clinician should change approaches so that individual goals may be addressed.

Hybrid Approaches

According to Fey (1986) **hybrid approaches** are attempts to develop intervention activities high in naturalness yet provide opportunities to work toward individualized goals. Hybrid approaches share three common characteristics: (1) the clinician develops individualized language goals; (2) the clinician selects materials and activities that are likely to elicit spontaneous utterances; and (3) the clinician modifies his or her own language not only to reflect the communication needs of the child but also to focus attention on the child's target forms.

Developing the Need to Communicate

The hybrid approaches are potentiated by the clinician's ability to create real needs to communicate. Fey (1986) described several procedures to help develop this need to communicate, including violating routine events, withholding objects, and violating the object's functions. To use **violating routine events**, the child and clinician have to share some routines so both have expectations. The routine may be as simple as rolling a ball back and forth. Once established, the clinician violates the routine by, for example, not rolling the ball to the child as expected but instead rolling the ball in the wrong direction. To use **withholding objects**, the clinician withholds an object that is needed for the activity. For example, the child is ready to start coloring. Everything is available: the chair, the table, the paper, but no crayons. The crayons are within the child's line of sight, but they are out of reach. To use **violating the object's function**, the clinician tries to use an object with an obvious function in the wrong way. For example, a routine has been established for preparing a bowl of Cheerios. The clinician is expected to fill the bowl with Cheerios. However, the bowl is placed upside down and the clinician gets ready to pour the cereal. All of these procedures have been designed to stimulate the child's need to communicate.

Varieties of Hybrid Approaches

Several forms of hybrid approaches to intervention, including focused stimulation, recasting, milieu teaching, dialogic book reading, and script training, are reviewed later. In **focused stimulation**, the clinician selects materials that encourage using target forms. The clinician provides repeated models of the target form in a meaningful communicative context. This aids the child's comprehension of that form and increases the likelihood that the child will imitate the target form. After modeling the target form, the clinician pauses and waits expectantly for a response. However, if the response does not occur spontaneously, it is neither prompted nor required. Various examples of the hybrid approach can be seen in Chapter 10 (exemplars 13, 16, 26, and 29).

When the child produces an utterance, the clinician may provide a recast. When **recasting**, the clinician responds to the child's utterance by using the correct form while maintaining its meaning (Proctor-Williams, Fey, & Loeb, 2001). Corrections are often grammatic or semantic but may include other linguistic parameters. In the recast, only the modified portion of the clinician's response is novel. Because the recast repeats some of the child's words, the correction minimizes the burden on the child's memory, which may enable the child to attend more fully to the modified portion. Moreover, the temporal proximity between the child's utterance and the recast may help make the corrective aspects of the recast apparent (Yoder, Spruytenburg, Edwards, & Davies, 1995). Recasts provide the child with a learning experience within a semantically and pragmatically appropriate context (Gillum, Camarata, Nelson, & Camarata, 2003), so the child does not have to acquire the form and learn its appropriate context as two distinct steps. Therefore, recasting in natural contexts facilitates generalization to other conversations. The recast serves as a model of a correct utterance, which the child is likely to imitate. However, recasts not only play a corrective role but also serve to provide a conversational turn. As such, recasts facilitate the flow of conversation and may be used with the CC approaches, as well as the hybrid approaches.

Recasts include expansions, extensions, and vertical restructuring. **Expansions** refer to responses to a child's spontaneous utterance, where the adult repeats some of the child's words and corrects the utterance by using a simple correct form as in (1).

1. Child: *Push car.*
    Adult: *Yes, you are pushing the car.*

Extensions are similar to expansions except that they go further by adding additional semantic detail as in (2).

2. Child: *Push car.*
    Adult: *Yes, you are pushing the car and it is going fast.*

As with recasts in general, expansions and extensions serve as models, and the child is likely to repeat them. **Vertical restructuring** is a particular form of expansion. However, it occurs over multiple turns. As shown in (3), the adult uses questions as conversational turns and then provides a model of the multiword utterance.

3. Adult: *Who is this?*
    Child: *Girl*
    Adult: *What is the girl throwing?*
    Child: *Ball*
    Adult: *Yes, the girl is throwing a ball.*

Milieu teaching is a general term that refers to applying operant conditioning principles in a quasi-natural setting. Specific variations include enhanced milieu teaching, incidental teaching, mand modeling, time delay, and prelinguistic milieu teaching. When milieu teaching is used in conjunction with environmental arranging and responsive interaction techniques, it is termed **enhanced milieu teaching** (EMT). Environmental arrangement and responsive interaction techniques were described under the CC approaches. However, with EMT, the adult also uses questions and prompts to elicit responding rather than simply relying on modeling.

Another variation of milieu teaching is incidental teaching. **Incidental teaching** is used throughout the day anytime a child initiates an interaction by specifying a reinforcer that an adult can satisfy. The adult uses the opportunity to focus attention on the child and to ask the child to elaborate on the topic before the reinforcement is delivered. The adult uses techniques such as modeling and prompting as well. The **mand-model** procedure is as an extension of incidental teaching (Peterson, 2004). To use it, the adult requests a verbal response from the child. If the response is correct, the adult provides intrinsic and extrinsic reinforcement. When the child's response is deficient, the adult provides a model of the target response and asks the child to repeat it. Because of the adult request for a verbal response, the mand-model procedure is useful with children who do not readily imitate. Time delay is another extension of incidental teaching (Peterson, 2004). In it, the adult uses **time delay**, or a strategic pause, to prompt the child to initiate. If the time delay is unsuccessful in eliciting a spontaneous vocal initiation, the adult may revert to the mand-model procedure.

Prelinguistic milieu teaching is yet another variation of the general milieu teaching model. However, it applies to young children who are neither using words nor exhibiting clear, frequent prelinguistic communication. The prelinguistic communicative skills, such as vocalizing, gesturing, gazing, and persisting in these behaviors, not only gets the message across to a responsive adult but also serves as a foundation for later language development.

Dialogic book reading promotes language development in language-impaired children. The idea is that the adult and child read the same book repeatedly so that their shared reading becomes a familiar routine. Books should reflect the child's developmental level and have good pictures to depict the story. As the adult reads the story, the child is encouraged to participate to the extent possible. Initially, the adult prompts the child to point to pictures describing the story. Later, the child answers questions about the story and the pictures. The adult recasts these responses and engages the child in dialogue about the story.

Gradually, the child assumes the greater burden of telling the story, while the adult's role is relegated to providing prompts and support.

Script training with language impairments is helpful because it primarily targets increasing social interactions and secondarily addresses lexical and grammatic forms. Often, 3- to 5-year-old children engage in **sociodramatic play**, or pretend play, with others using reciprocal roles embedded in themes, for example, parent–child, doctor–patient, salesperson–customer and so on. Children's successful engagement in such play reflects their cognitive framework for understanding the themes, as well as the concomitant roles and language. This cognitive framework is called **script**. Each time children participate in a particular theme, their script is enriched. The typically developing child acquires a wide range of scripts that are called on for sociodramatic play and serve as a foundation for more advanced social interactions. However, some language-impaired children lack this background. Consequently, they may be unsuccessful in playing with peers and unprepared for more advanced social exchanges.

In script training, the child engages in social interactions around particular themes. Therefore, props are provided to support whatever theme has been selected, for example, playing house, which may involve the use of dolls, doll clothes, and doll beds. The language-impaired child engages in this activity in dyads, with a language-normal peer or with the clinician. The clinician models the behavior, which is then imitated and rehearsed by the children in play. The clinician also employs prompts. Models and prompts are faded with skill acquisition. As children acquire skills of interacting in the context of a particular theme, they also acquire the language appropriate to the script. Planning a series of different scripts is helpful.

School-aged children are expected to engage in conversations with peers and others. Nippold (2000) showed that as grade level increases, the students' conversational skills increase in a systematic fashion. However, language-impaired students often do not possess the same proficiency in conversational skills as their language-normal peers (Paul, 2007). Therefore, conversational skills, such as maintaining topic, turn-taking, requesting clarification, and repairing conversations are important treatment targets for language-impaired school-aged children.

These conversational skills, collectively referred to as **conversational discourse**, may be taught following the script-training model in dyads using language-normal peers or a clinician. Either way, the clinician models the appropriate conversational skill in conversational contexts and asks the student to imitate the skill. During the student's imitation, the clinician uses models and prompts as necessary to elicit the target response. Then, as the student acquires the skill, the models and prompts are faded. Following acquisition, the clinician asks the student to apply the new skill in conversations with peers. The student reports back periodically on these experiences, and the clinician listens and provides advice and encouragement.

Personal narratives are a form of discourse for telling others a story about oneself. **Narrative discourse** differs from conversational discourse in important ways. Narratives tend to be monologues, but conversations tend to be dialogues. Narratives are also more structured than conversations. The storyteller is expected to progress from beginning to end in a coherent fashion. Telling personal narratives is important in life because it is a mechanism for explaining oneself to others. However, language-impaired schoolchildren tend to be deficient in this important skill (McCabe & Rollins, 1994). Therefore, telling personal narratives represents an important treatment target for these students.

Storytelling skills may be taught using script training. To do so, the clinician starts by eliciting a story from the student. To elicit a story, the clinician should model telling a brief story. Peterson and McCabe (1983) indicated that children most readily talk about injuries, so that is a good place to start. The clinician says something like, "I hurt my finger fixing the door. Did you ever hurt yourself? I'll tell you my story, and then you tell me your story." The clinician should elicit and record about three stories to assess the child's narrative skills.

McCabe and Bliss (2003) developed the Narrative Assessment Profile (NAP) to evaluate narrative coherence. The NAP consists of six dimensions: (1) topic maintenance, whether all utterances relate to the topic; (2) event sequencing, whether the events are logically sequenced; (3) informativeness, whether there is sufficient detail; (4) referencing, whether there is adequate identification of individuals, locations, and features; (5) conjunctive cohesion, whether the words (such as *then*, *because*, *so*, *but*) link the events together; and (6) fluency, whether there is sufficient momentum to the spoken presentation that the story makes sense. The clinician evaluates each dimension of the student's stories to prepare to start script training.

The clinician tells a story as a means of eliciting a story. First, the clinician draws the story to be told using stick-figure drawings. Then, the clinician models telling the story, using the drawings as prompts. Similarly, when the student tells his or her story, he or she first draws it and uses the pictures as prompts. During the student's narrative, the clinician provides verbal prompts, including *wh-* questions to help the student address deficiencies in story cohesion. The clinician should focus on only one dimension at a time to avoid overwhelming the student. Furthermore, priority should be given to the first three dimensions of the NAP because they are more basic. At any rate, this sequence of modeling by the clinician and imitation by the student is repeated, and through this rehearsal process, the student acquires the script, or framework, for telling personal stories. As the storytelling skill is acquired, the models and prompts are faded. Then, the clinician should collaborate with the teacher to devise a classroom assignment in which narrative skills can be practiced in the natural context of the classroom.

Levels of Intervention

Intervention in child-language disorders occurs at different levels: acquisition, maintenance, and generalization. Reflecting on levels of intervention may help the clinician focus treatment with more precision. The term **acquisition** designates the initial learning of the linguistic skill. For example, a clinician may train a toddler to name common objects through modeling the correct label. After a period of time, the toddler begins to label these objects during training, indicating that acquisition is occurring.

It is hoped that language forms, once acquired, continue. However, without a maintaining experience, they may be lost (Olswang & Bain, 1991). Following acquisition, there is a need to determine whether the forms have been preserved or **maintained**. If not, then the need for a maintenance program or a review of previously acquired forms is indicated.

The term **generalization** refers to the occurrence of a behavior in contexts in which it has never been trained. As described by Stokes and Baer (1977) in their classic article, generalization may be promoted by several techniques. These techniques were designated as a technology of generalization and included train and hope, sequential modification, introduce naturally maintaining contingencies, program common stimuli, and mediate generalization, which are described next. These techniques may be implemented during treatment or as a follow-up to treatment.

The technology of generalization has been extensively applied in communication disorders (McReynolds & Spradlin, 1989). Train and hope dramatizes the notion that clinicians often neglect the important consideration of generalization. Although generalization on its own is indeed possible, the clinician should at least check. When generalization is not seen, then procedures may be employed to train the target response in each environment where it is lacking. This technique to facilitating generalization is called **sequential modification**. Another technique is to **introduce naturally maintaining contingencies** by selecting training target responses likely to receive intrinsic reinforcement. For example, if a child is taught to request juice, making such a request is likely to result in the child obtaining the juice, which promotes the general use of requesting as a response class. In **program common stimuli,** salient elements from the natural communicative environment are brought into the treatment room. For example, bringing the child's peers into treatment sessions may facilitate generalization of skills to conversations with them in the natural environment. Finally, a child may be taught to **mediate generalization**. This technique is relevant for children with sufficient cognitive resources. The clinician teaches the child the rule for applying a certain behavior and then relies on his or her self-management skills to do so. For example, a child may be taught the rule, "When you see a friend for the first time in the day, greet that person."

Chapter Summary

In this chapter, intervention is presented conceptually. A continuum of naturalness is used to describe a wide range of eclectic treatment approaches, including clinician directed at the low end, client centered at the high end, and hybrid intermediately. Variables to be manipulated, associated with each treatment approach, are defined. Finally, intervention levels are described, including acquisition, maintenance, and generalization as a means of adding precision and specificity to the intervention process.

Terms from the Chapter

Acquisition *(104)*

Child-centered approaches *(97)*

Clinician-directed approaches *(95)*

Continuum of naturalness *(94)*

Conversational discourse *(102)*

Dependent variable *(93)*

Dialogic book reading *(101)*

Discrete trials *(95)*

Enhanced milieu teaching *(101)*

Expansions *(100)*

Extensions *(100)*

Extrinsic reinforcement *(95)*

Facilitative play *(97)*
Fading *(95)*
Feedback *(95)*
Figurative language *(96)*
Focused stimulation *(99)*
General stimulation *(97)*
Generalization *(104)*
Hybrid approaches *(98)*
Hypothesis testing *(93)*
Incidental teaching *(101)*
Independent variable *(93)*
Intrinsic reinforcement *(95)*
Introduce naturally maintaining
    contingencies *(105)*
Maintenance *(104)*
Mand-model *(101)*
Mediate generalization *(105)*
Metalinguistic ability *(96)*
Metaphor *(96)*
Milieu teaching *(100)*
Model *(95)*

Narrative discourse *(103)*
Personal narrative *(103)*
Prelinguistic milieu teaching *(101)*
Program common stimuli *(105)*
Prompt *(95)*
Recasting *(99)*
Reinforcement *(95)*
Script *(102)*
Script training *(102)*
Sequential modification *(105)*
Shaping *(95)*
Sociodramatic play *(102)*
Target response *(95)*
Therapeutic register *(94)*
Time delay *(101)*
Training stimuli *(95)*
Vertical restructuring *(100)*
Violating object's function *(99)*
Violating routine events *(99)*
Withholding objects *(99)*

References

Fey, M. E. (1986). *Language intervention with young children*. San Diego, CA:
    College Hill Press.

Gillum, H., Camarata, S., Nelson, K., & Camarata, M. (2003). A comparison
    of natural and analog treatment effects in children with expressive language
    disorders and poor preintervention imitation skills. *Journal of Positive Behavior
    Interventions, 5*, 171–178.

Hegde, M. N. (1994). *Clinical research in communication disorders: Principles and
    strategies* (2nd ed.). Austin, TX: PRO-ED.

Hepting, N. H., & Goldstein, H. (1996). What's natural about naturalistic lan-
    guage intervention. *Journal of Early Intervention, 20*, 249–265.

Hubbell, R. (1981). *Children's language disorders: An integrated approach*. Engle-
    wood Cliffs, NJ: Prentice Hall.

McCabe, A., & Bliss, L. S. (2003). *Patterns of narrative discourse: A multicultural,
    life span approach*. Boston, MA: Pearson Education.

McCabe, A., & Rollins, P. R. (1994). Assessment of preschool narrative skills.
    American Journal of Speech-Language Pathology, A Journal of Clinical Practice, 3,
    45–56.

McReynolds, L. V., & Spradlin, J. E. (Eds.). (1989). *Generalization strategies in
    the treatment of communication disorders*. Toronto, Canada: B.C. Decker.

Nippold, M. A. (2000). Language development during adolescent years: Aspects of pragmatics, syntax and semantics. *Topics in Language Disorders, 20,* 15–28.

Olswang, L., & Bain, B. (1991). Intervention issues for toddlers with specific language impairments. *Topics in Language Disorders, 11,* 69–86.

Paul, R. (2007). *Language disorders from infancy through adolescence: Assessment and intervention* (3rd ed.). St. Louis: Mosby.

Peterson, C., & McCabe, A. (1983). *Developmental psycholinguistics: Three ways of looking at a child's narrative.* New York, NY: Plenum Press.

Peterson, P. (2004). Naturalistic language teaching procedures for children at risk for language delay. *Behavior Analyst Today, 5,* 404–424.

Proctor-Williams, K., Fey, M., & Loeb, D. (2001). Parental recasts and production of copulas and articles by children with specific language impairment and typical language. *Journal of Speech-Language Pathology, 10,* 155–168.

Sheng, L., McGregor, K. K., & Xu, Y. (2003). Prosodic and lexical-syntactic aspects of the therapeutic register. *Clinical Linguistics and Phonetics, 17,* 355–363.

Stokes, T. F., & Baer, D. M. (1977). An implicit technology of generalization. *Journal of Applied Behavior Analysis, 10,* 349–367.

Wallach, G. P., & Miller, L. (1988). *Language intervention and academic success.* Boston, MA: Little, Brown.

Yoder, J., Spruytenburg, H., Edwards, A., & Davies, B. (1995). Effects of verbal routine contexts and expansions on gains in mean length of utterance in children with developmental delays. *Language, Speech and Hearing Services in Schools, 26,* 21–32.

C H A P T E R   7

Augmentative/Alternative Communication

Lizbeth Curme Stevens

Chapter Objectives

After reading this chapter, you should be able to:

- Define augmentative and alternative communication (AAC) and describe its components (i.e., symbols, strategies, aids, and techniques).
- Identify types of children who may benefit from AAC.
- Explain guiding principles for best practice in AAC.
- Discuss assessment procedures for determining appropriate symbols, strategies, aids, and techniques for enhanced communication.
- Discuss how to implement AAC for children with severe communication impairments.

In the introductory chapter, a framework for the process of communication was presented (Denes & Pinson, 1993). Communication involves an exchange of information between individuals. This may be accomplished through various ways, including but not limited to speaking, writing, gesturing, using facial expressions, and body language. For some individuals, using these conventional means of communication is not possible. This chapter explores alternatives available for children with severe communication disorders.

Augmentative/Alternative Communication

Augmentative/alternative communication (**AAC**) is "the practice of using compensatory treatments to supplement or replace natural speech and writing" (Ogletree & Oren, 2006, p. ix). More broadly,

AAC is considered a multidisciplinary field of research and clinical or educational practice whose stakeholders explore and apply information to support individuals unable to meet daily communication demands in conventional ways (e.g., through speech, gestures, and writing) (ASHA, 2005; Beukelman & Mirenda, 2005). People with severe communication disorders of expression or comprehension may be supported in both oral and written modalities.

Specifically, AAC may be conceptualized as an integrated system of four components: (1) symbols, (2) aids, (3) strategies, and (4) techniques (ASHA, 2004). Brief descriptions of these terms, as they relate to AAC, follow with elaboration in the assessment and intervention sections:

Symbol. A symbol stands for or represents something else. It may be a visual, auditory, or other (e.g., tactile) representation. For example, hearing your mother announce "Dinner!" conveys a call to the table for food. Likewise, seeing the McDonald's golden arches atop a building indicates that food awaits you therein. Symbols include both spoken and written words, braille, signs, objects, miniatures, pictures, photos, and gestures. Symbols may be **aided** (i.e., requiring external assistance or equipment to produce as in pictures, objects, and braille) or **unaided** (i.e., produced on or with the body such as sign and speech).

Aid. An aid is an object or device, either electronic or nonelectronic, used to transmit or receive messages. Examples of **low technology** (**low-tech**) aids are communication books, boards, or wallets and eye-gaze frames. **High technology** (**high-tech**) aids include **speech generating devices** (SGDs; also known as **voice output communication aids**, or **VOCAs**) and computers outfitted with special software. Some systems of communication that use no aid at all (i.e., unaided) include speech and sign. These are examples of **no-tech** (i.e., absence of any technology) solutions.

Strategy. A strategy conveys messages in the most efficient and effective manner. Individuals may adopt specific strategies to enhance their communication. In general, the three purposes of strategies are to improve (1) timing of messages, (2) grammar of composed messages, and (3) rate of communication.

Technique. A technique is a method for transmitting information. When we use words or signs, we transmit information by the techniques of speaking and signing, respectively. Children unable to speak might use a physical aid of some type to communicate (e.g., a **communication board** or an electronic device that speaks). In such cases, the techniques employed are **direct selection** (e.g., pointing to a picture or word on the board) or **scanning** (e.g., using special software and switches with the SGD in which choices are presented automatically to the child who selects the desired message by depressing a switch when it appears). As demonstrated, techniques may or may not use a physical aid.

In sum, although AAC includes the previous components, it remains an integrated system. For optimal communication, all components of the system should be in synergy with one another. Although components may be addressed separately, the gestalt should be considered. For example, a compensatory approach with some individuals unable to speak or write may be to equip them with a computer or electronic device that speaks or types. Although this technology may support the process of communication, it alone is not considered AAC. The device is not the end goal, rather, it is the means to the end, successful communication.

As noted previously, we all communicate in various ways using many different types of symbols. In intervention, the goal must be to empower the child to communicate independently with all of his or her residual abilities combined with added supports determined to enhance communication. In many instances, there may not be a single AAC system used by an individual but a number of different ones, depending on the context (Cumley, Maro, & Stanek, 2009).

Who Uses Augmentative/Alternative Communication?

Children who use AAC compose a heterogeneous group. Impairments that prevent them from speaking or writing may be either congenital or acquired. Different types include cognitive, sensory, neurological, and emotional impairments (Musselwhite & St. Louis, 1986). For example, children with autism, cerebral palsy, or cognitive impairment (e.g., resulting from Down, Prader-Willi, or Angelman's syndrome) may benefit from AAC to optimize communication. Likewise, children with acquired injuries (e.g., a traumatic brain injury sustained in a motor vehicle accident or spinal cord paralysis from a diving accident) may also use either temporary or permanent AAC support. Clearly, there is no one typical AAC user. Children with diverse diagnoses are all potential candidates for AAC to improve their expression and comprehension both in speaking and in writing.

People communicate in various ways symbolically, as well as nonsymbolically. Furthermore, not all communication is necessarily intentional. In the broadest sense then, everyone can and does communicate.

Therefore, all individuals, whether they communicate deliberately or not and whether they communicate symbolically (e.g., with words) or not (e.g., through a stiffening of their body as a negative response to a stimulus) are potential beneficiaries of AAC. There are then no prerequisites for eligibility to receive AAC supports (Baumgart, Johnson, & Helmstetter, 1990).

However, while all children may benefit from communication facilitation through AAC, selection of the appropriate system clearly depends on the individual child's needs and capabilities, including his or her current level of language or symbol usage. Purchase of an expensive, electronic, state-of-the-art communication device will not ensure success for the child if she or he is unable to use it (Calculator, 2000). Consequently, choice of a system should reflect that which will be most effectively learned and implemented with the child.

Guiding Principles for Best Practice in Augmentative/Alternative Communication

AAC has been described as a multidisciplinary field. The knowledge and skills required of speech-language pathologists (SLPs) for the area of practice are formidable (ASHA, 2002; 2004; 2005). The underlying principles for implementing exemplary AAC practices in both assessment and intervention follow:

1. *Respect rights of child and family*: Although early implementation of AAC is optimal, the choices of the family and child must be honored. Forming a partnership with the parents may be most important to moving the child's language and communication skills forward. Frequently, parents view the recommendation of AAC as a last resort, synonymous with abandonment of speech. Be prepared to enlighten families about the value of enhancing communication skills to build language necessary for developing literacy. Inform others about the evidence that AAC does not interfere with the development of speech but may facilitate it (Millar, Light, & Schlosser, 2006).

2. *Educate others*: Empower the child who uses AAC and his or her family with tools and resources to take charge of the system: its implementation, training, and expansion. Facilitate their skill development so that they may teach others about AAC and the child's unique system as she or he interacts with others. Spend intervention time not only in working directly with the child and

family but also in training all communication partners to ensure that desired strategies may be implemented when you are not present. View this as equally important to the time you spend with the child, as you are enabling others to advance the child's skills far beyond what you alone could do.

3. *Achieve more through teamwork*: Teamwork is critical to success in AAC. No one person can know all that is required for effective AAC support. The family and child are at the core of the team. Other stakeholders may include the teacher, SLP, and other professionals (e.g., assistive technology specialist, occupational therapist [OT], physical therapist [PT], and psychologist) and paraprofessionals. Determine persons best suited to assist in assessing and instructing the child. Input from everyone is essential for effective intervention (Beukelman & Mirenda, 2005). Although team membership and leadership may change over time, the child and parents remain constant. Remember that *together everyone achieves more* (i.e., T-E-A-M).

4. *Consider multiple modalities/symbols*: Routinely incorporate multiple communication strategies and goals (retaining speech or vocalizations) as appropriate. More than one communication system may need to be selected, and effective implementation of AAC often depends on context and communication partner. Flexibility is important for optimal outcomes.

5. *Recognize change as a constant*: For many children, using AAC may last a lifetime, given their developmental growth, as well as advances in technology. Consequently, assessment and intervention will be ongoing. Routine review of the communication system(s), including aids and strategies, will be necessary at regularly scheduled intervals.

6. *Focus on capability*: Enhancing communication requires using the individual's strengths. What the child is unable to do is clearly apparent. Consequently, the key to unlocking communication potential through AAC is to focus on what is possible. Keen observation by team members, willingness to explore many avenues for communication, perseverance, and dedication to the outcome are requirements for success.

7. *Establish meaningful goals*: Obtain input from the child, family, and teacher about the most important and compelling communication needs. Successful AAC provision is not measured, for example, by how many different signs a child knows or can produce in a

therapy session but by his or her appropriate functional communication (e.g., using a sign in daily situations). Regularly reevaluate communication targets and progress toward them. Ensure that facilitation toward meeting these targets is provided in real contexts for optimal success.

Assessment for Augmentative/Alternative Communication

The AAC assessment process entails examining the child's existing communication, determining his or her abilities, and finally selecting the AAC system(s) based on this information. Assessing children with severe communication disorders that prevent them from fully participating in daily activities is a challenging task. Even though all nonspeaking children are candidates for AAC, they require different supports, depending on individual needs. Such needs are determined through the assessment process, which may be adapted to address specific areas (Shipley & McAfeey, 2009).

Assessment begins with a thorough understanding of how the child presently communicates. This requires both observing the child and interviewing many individuals who know the child well. At the same time, it is necessary to gather information about the child's capability through observation, interviews, and testing. Once this information has been gathered, the final phase of the assessment, selection of an appropriate communication system (or systems) may be undertaken. Although many options are available, both electronic and nonelectronic (i.e., high and low tech and even no tech, as in the selection of sign), the child's individual needs and capabilities must be the primary determiners in the selection process. This process has been described as matching the features of the system (or aid) to the needs and ability of the child (Glennen & DeCoste, 1997). Assessment for children who require AAC support can never be a single event; moreover, as children grow in their use of the chosen system(s), adjustments may be necessary. Therefore, assessment is a continuing and ongoing process.

Team Approach

As identified in the guiding principles, a team approach works best. No one individual should do the AAC assessment alone. For example, while the SLP may know the most about language and communication, the family may best understand the child's needs, and the teacher may best understand his or her capabilities. An assistive technology specialist may be the expert resource on suitable technology. Each team member has a role to play in gathering information for decision making about which AAC system is best. Depending on the unique needs of the child and available resources, team configurations may vary.

Collecting Information

Gathering data for the assessment will involve interviews, observations, and testing by the team. Required information for all assessments includes (1) background information, including medical and educational history with reference to any previous use of AAC (i.e., case history); (2) description of all ways the child currently communicates, including details on frequency, partners, and effectiveness; (3) determination of the child's cognitive abilities, including memory and reasoning skills, as well as exploring symbolic representation; (4) determining the child's language ability (i.e., semantic, syntactic, pragmatic) for both comprehension and expression in both oral and written modalities; (5) review of child's behavior, which relates to communication and level of intentionality (if the child communicates nonsymbolically). Other information as needed on an individual case-by-case basis may include: assessment of motor, perceptual, and sensory systems by the appropriate professional (e.g., occupational therapist) affecting the child's ability to access AAC. In addition, assessment for seating and positioning is critical for children who have a diagnosed medical condition (e.g., cerebral palsy) that may affect their ability to access symbols (Baumgart, Johnson, & Helmstetter, 1990; Calculator, 2000). Only a few standardized protocols exist for conducting assessments for AAC. None are comprehensive. A useful approach to assess and implement assistive technology, the SETT framework, may be helpful in structuring AAC intervention (Zabala, 1995).

Selecting a System

The choice of a system (i.e., the gestalt, which encompasses symbols, techniques, aids, and strategies) is based on careful comparison of the collected assessment information (i.e., the child's needs, current communication methods, and capabilities) and the characteristics or features of systems. Routinely, a system should be tried out for best fit. In other words, precise determination of the optimal match for a child may take time, in which one or more approaches or aids are explored. Particularly, if an electronic device is selected, a trial period is advisable before purchase. In other words, unlike many assessments completed at one point in time, an AAC assessment typically requires multiple sessions over a period of days, weeks, or even months if trials of several devices/aids are involved. Using AAC entails ongoing maintenance and oversight. It is a continuous process. Furthermore, assessment needs to recur simply because, as the child grows and develops (both cognitively and linguistically), there may be a need to adapt the AAC system.

As mentioned previously in the guidelines, multiple communication modes and symbols are the norm, rather than the exception for all individuals. Consequently, the child with a severe communication impairment likewise must be supported to communicate in various ways, with different systems across contexts. It would not be unusual then to have a child who uses signs with his or her parents at home but employs a combination of familiar signs with a communication book in school.

In some instances, a particular system may be chosen immediately to fulfill a unique need or purpose. For example, a specific low-tech approach might be implemented if a child is self-injurious. The system might later be expanded or replaced to include voice output when the child's behavior has stabilized.

Assessment Specifics: Exploring Language and Symbolization Skills

Gestures/Signs

Considerations in selecting gestures or signs as a communication mode include the child's motor and imitative skills. However, inability to imitate does not preclude this symbol choice since gesture and sign may be taught through hand-shaping practices. If the child already uses some idiosyncratic movements to convey meaning (e.g., covering face with hands to signal rejection), these behaviors may be shaped and replaced by more conventional communication gestures and signs.

Visual Symbols

Symbol assessment is accomplished in numerous steps (Beukelman & Mirenda, 2005; Glennen & DeCoste, 1997). To begin, collect about 10 functional items that the child knows and recognizes. Next assemble various symbols depicting these (e.g., color or black and white photographs, line drawings, miniatures).

Step 1. *Functional use*: Present the child with the items one at a time to see whether he or she can use them functionally. If the child is physically unable to do this, you may model various behaviors to the child and confirm with him or her that the use is appropriate.

Step 2. *Receptive label*: Present the child with two or more symbols (for each item) and ask him or her to select the symbol that matches the named item. You can assess multiple types of symbols in this way. If the child does not know the label or name, use an alternative procedure: visual matching. Present child with an object and two or more labels and ask him or her to select the symbol that best matches the object. Or present the child with a symbol and two or more objects and ask him or her to select the object that best matches the symbol.

Step 3. *Contextual use*: Next evaluate symbol use to communicate:

Question–answer format: Present the child with an array of various symbols and ask general questions (e.g., *What do you eat for breakfast?*).

Natural format: In a real situation, such as snack time, provide child with symbols and prompt a request (e.g., *I don't know what you want. Can you help me out?*).

Step 4. *Advanced symbol use*: This procedure may be used to determine the child's capability to use more than one symbol in succession, as well as symbols that represent concepts other than nouns. Use a display for a game (e.g., *go fish*) with symbols depicting nouns (e.g., *ace*), verb forms (e.g., *go fish*), and so on. Model display use and see whether the child can produce or reproduce this behavior.

Step 5. *Symbol categorization and association*: Have the child sort symbols from two or more categories (e.g., food, transportation, and clothing).

Step 6. *Determination of symbol(s)*: After assessing the child's symbolic abilities, you may be able to discern his or her level of current symbol usage and preference. For children who are unable to accomplish step 1, you may need to implement strategies for "beginning communicators," which support the child in developing cause and effect, understanding awareness of preferences, and teaching functional communication skills and the association of symbols and their referents. For children with the ability to use symbols, the type selected is based on the preceding assessment procedure. Easy-to-learn and use symbols are preferable. Instruction on more complex symbol types may also be undertaken; however, the set selected first must be immediately accessible with minimum effort.

Language Assessment

The team will gather information relative to the child's language skills early in the assessment process. Although giving standardized instruments may be useful, adaptations might be required for administration, thus disqualifying the scores as "standard." However, it is important to secure approximations of receptive language level for symbol selection and training. Language tests that require a "yes" or "no" response or a multiple-choice format are preferred. Suggested tests used for this purpose include the PPVT (4th edition) (Dunn, Dunn, Williams, & Wang, 2007), the MacArthur Communicative Developmental Inventories (CDI; Fenson, Dale, Reznick, et al., 1992, the Sequenced Inventory of Communication Development-Revised (SICD) (Hedrick, Prather, & Tobin, 1984), and the Bracken Basic Concept Scale-Revised (Bracken, 1998).

Intervention

Implementation of AAC for children with severe communication impairments is something that is likely to co-occur with the ongoing assessment process. Determining the most appropriate symbols, techniques, strategies, and aid (if applicable) will likely require the team to be involved in various activities for trial periods in which specific skills are targeted. The guidelines for best practice apply to the intervention phase, as well as assessment. To recap, intervention through a team effort in which the child and family are central should focus on long- and short-term goals using multiple modalities and symbols. The ultimate objective is the child's meaningful participation in daily life activities through effective communication. Considerable effort should be expended in training the child, parents, and team in using the system in addition to educating all communication partners on how to support and enhance the child's communication.

Specific suggestions for communication partners follow:

1. Do not talk for the child who has the necessary AAC tools; give him or her an opportunity to interact with others and to respond

to questions or initiate conversation first without any assistance; peers (vs. adults) frequently make the best partners.

2. Adjust your communication style to allow more pause time for the child's responses; refrain from repeating your message during this time (e.g., ask only one question at a time); learn to pause and wait; allow extra time for the child to respond as needed.

3. Allow the child to experience communication breakdowns and the opportunity to fix them; do not always jump in to save the day, but remember that the goal is to support the child's independent communication by teaching him or her how to resolve problems.

4. To facilitate the child's participation in group discussions, ask the child multiple-choice questions; however, do not limit the child's opportunities by putting him or her only in a respondent role (i.e., answering questions); alternatively, give the child an opportunity to prepare his or her message in advance by giving him or her the question you will ask.

5. Encourage the child to use multiple modes of communication (including gestures, facial expressions, and eye gaze), along with the AAC; respond to any, and do not insist that the child use the device if a head nod is sufficient.

6. Promote conversation by commenting yourself and then pausing (e.g., *I love my new school*) versus asking a question (e.g., *Do you like school?*) to increase language usage and support independence in communication; recognize that the child will not improve in expressive ability if he or she only has an opportunity to respond to *wh-* or *yes/no* questions.

Additional general suggestions for AAC implementation are as follows:

1. Provide augmented input to children with poor receptive language by using symbols selected not only for output or expression alone but also for input. For example, if the child is being taught sign to communicate expressively, then routinely sign to the child along with talking as a model. Do the same with picture symbols. Point to symbols as you speak the word.

2. Create opportunities for the child to communicate successfully in meaningful and motivating contexts. In other words, AAC support and instruction should occur throughout the day, not just at specific therapy times. For example, enable the child to choose an ice cream dessert for a school lunch if this is an option. Start first

with communication activities that interest the child, not necessarily activities that are important to the teacher (e.g., signaling to use the bathroom). Regularly ask the child (or parents) to verify importance.

3. Select age-appropriate vocabulary and activities so that the child may readily interact with peers.

4. Enlist the child's peers to become communication partners to facilitate the child's communication in the classroom. If the child is using a voice output device with digitized (i.e., human/recorded) speech, consider using the voice of a peer for messages. Peers may also assist in programming devices and selecting age-appropriate vocabulary.

5. Target messages to be used that are functional. In other words, select vocabulary likely to be elicited during the day and for which another might need to respond for the child if the child cannot.

6. Involve the child in selecting symbols and arranging them when creating low-tech communication displays; attempt to use the display yourself first or have the child's peers do so to make certain that you have included all that is necessary in that particular context. Remember that the child may be unable to participate unless he or she has the appropriate vocabulary.

7. Recognize that to replace existing maladaptive communication behaviors (e.g., head banging to get attention) the new communication system must be as efficient as or more efficient than the existing one.

8. Provide the child with a signaling device (e.g., bell or buzzer) independent of the child's communication system, especially if it is low tech, so that he or she can capture someone's attention, particularly if the child is unable to move.

Chapter Summary

Augmentative/alternative communication (AAC) is defined, and its components (i.e., symbols, techniques, aids, and strategies) are described. Children with severe expressive and receptive communication disorders who might benefit from AAC are identified. Principles for best practice are outlined with specific suggestions for assessment and intervention. Tools and resources are provided that will support the selection of appropriate system(s) to enhancing the communication skills of these children.

Terms from the Chapter

Aid *(110)*
Aided symbol *(110)*
Augmentative/alternative
  communication (AAC) *(109)*
Communication board *(110)*
Direct selection *(110)*
High technology (high tech) *(110)*
Low technology (low tech) *(110)*
No tech systems *(110)*

Scanning *(111)*
Speech generating device
  (SGD) *(110)*
Strategy *(110)*
Symbol *(110)*
Technique *(110)*
Unaided symbol *(110)*
Voice output communication
  aid (VOCA) *(110)*

References

American Speech-Language-Hearing Association. (2002). *Augmentative and alternative communication: Knowledge and skills for service delivery* [knowledge and skills]. Retrieved from www.asha.org/policy

American Speech-Language-Hearing Association. (2004). *Roles and responsibilities of speech-language pathologists with respect to augmentative and alternative communication: Technical report* [technical report]. Retrieved from www.asha.org/policy

American Speech-Language-Hearing Association. (2005). *Roles and responsibilities of speech-language pathologists with respect to augmentative and alternative communication: Position statement* [position statement]. Retrieved from www.asha.org/policy

Baumgart, D., Johnson, J., & Helmstetter, E. (1990). *Augmentative and alternative communication systems for persons with moderate and severe disabilities.* Baltimore, MD: Paul H. Brookes.

Beukelman, D., & Mirenda, P. (2005). *Augmentative and alternative communication: Supporting children and adults with complex communication needs* (3rd ed.). Baltimore, MD: Paul H. Brookes.

Bracken, B. (1998). Bracken basic concept scale-revised. San Antonio, TX: Psych. Corp.

Calculator, S. N. (2000). Augmentative and alternative communication. In E. P. Dodge (Ed.), *The survival guide for school-based speech-language pathologists* (pp. 345–363). San Diego, CA: Singular.

Cumley, J., Maro, J., & Stanek, M. (2009). Assistive technology for communication. In J. Gierach (Ed.), *Assessing students need for assistive technology* (5th ed.). Wisconsin Assistive Technology Institute. Retrieved from www.wati.org

Denes, P. B., & Pinson, E. N. (1993). *The speech chain: The physics and biology of spoken language.* New York, NY: W. H. Freeman.

Dunn, L., Dunn, L., Williams, K., & Wang, J. (2007). *Peabody picture vocabulary test (PPVT)* (4th edition). Circle Pines, MN: AGS.

Fenson, L., Dale, D., Reznick, J., Thal, D., Bates, E., Hartwig, M., . . . Reilly, J. (1992). *MacArthur communicative developmental inventories (CDI).* Baltimore, MD: Paul H. Brookes.

Glennen, S., & DeCoste, D. (1997). *Handbook of augmentative and alternative communication*. San Diego, CA: Singular.

Hedrick, D., Prather, E., & Tobin, A. (1984). *Sequenced inventory of communicative development (SICD)*. Seattle: University of Washington Press.

Millar, D. C., Light, J. C., & Schlosser, R. W. (2006). The impact of augmentative and alternative communication intervention on the speech production of individuals with developmental disabilities: A research review. *Journal of Speech, Language, and Hearing Research, 49*, 248–264.

Musselwhite, C., & St. Louis, K. (1988). *Communication programming for persons with severe handicaps* (2nd ed.). Austin, TX: PRO-ED.

Ogletree, B. T., & Oren, T. (2006). *How to use augmentative and alternative communication*. Austin, TX: PRO-ED.

Shipley, K., & McAfee, J. (2009). *Assessment in speech-language pathology* (4th ed.). Clifton Park, NY: Delmar Learning.

Zabala, J. (1995, October). *The SETT framework: Critical areas to consider when making informed assistive technology decision*. Presentation at Closing the Gap Conference, Minneapolis, MN.

Evaluation Resources Specifically Developed for AAC

The Nonspeech Test for Receptive/Expressive Language (Huer, 1988)—Don Johnston Developmental Equipment, Inc.

Interaction Checklist for Augmentative Communication (INCH) (Revised) (Bolton and Dashiel, 1991)—Imaginart

www.dougdodgen.com
    Commercial feature match software available to assist in AAC assessment process targeting school-age children and adults

www.augcomm.com/needsfirst.html
    Needs First: AugCom System Search Tool, developed by Barbara Couse Adams and Cindy L. George (this is for target population of school-age children). Web site provides a link to all current AAC devices and commercial software that will match child's capabilities to available technology.

Recommended Internet Resources

http://www.aacinstitute.org
    Affiliated with Edinborough University of Pennsylvania and includes information on AAC and resources for students, professionals, and consumers, including parents. Lists of training institutions, research, and evidence-based practice. Offers free continuing education units (CEUs) for several online courses.

http://www.aac-rerc.com
>   Rehabilitation Engineering and Research Center in Communication Enhancement is a collaborative funded by a grant from NIDRR (National Institute on Disability and Rehabilitation Research) in the U.S. Department of Education's Office of Special Education and Rehabilitative Services (OSERS). Includes Web casts on various topics and numerous resources and publications.

http://www.aacintervention.com
>   Site of Dr. Caroline Musselwhite; commercial products to aid in making overlays for early intervention with AAC; also gives helpful information on how to begin using AAC with a nonspeaking child; features local and national presentations/conference dates, and tips of the month.

http://aac.unl.edu
>   University of Nebraska-Lincoln has information, including AAC device tutorials, definitions of AAC glossary under "Academic" page, frequently used vocabulary lists for different age groups and many other resources.

http://www.communicationmatrix.org
>   A widely used instrument by Charity Rowland available free to parents online, which assists in determining the communication skills of very young children or those who are just beginning to communicate.

http://www.augcominc.com/newsletters/?fuseaction=newsletters
>   Past issues of 124 newsletters of *Augmentative Communication News* and *Alternatively Speaking*, published by Sarah Blackstone, a leader in the field of AAC, are now available at no cost.

http://www.lburkhart.com/sr.htm
>   Selected vendors and manufacturers with annotations/descriptions of products. Articles and presentations presented by Linda Burkhart concerning support for young children who need AAC, including topics of partner-assisted scanning, switch construction, and support for children with autism.

http://www.unl.edu/yaack/
>   Augmentative Alternative Communication (AAC) Connecting Young Kids. Site providing information concerning children and AAC devices, such as when and where to secure help regarding AAC; information on how to choose the best AAC system, etc.

www.vantatenhove.com
>   Gail VanTatenhove's Web site, which has free materials, including vocabulary lists of adults, elders, and young children, as well as a client vocabulary checklist

www.wati.org
>   Wisconsin's assistive technology institute. Many free materials to support assistive technology (AT) with various types of student. Includes downloadable handbook on AT, including a chapter on AAC.

AUGMENTATIVE/ALTERNATIVE COMMUNICATION

CHAPTER 8

Multicultural Issues in Assessment and Intervention

Ana Claudia Harten

Chapter Objectives

After reading this chapter, you should be able to:

- Differentiate between language differences and language-learning disability.
- Discuss cultural differences that affect children's communication behaviors.
- Describe some typical behaviors associated with bilingual development.
- Identify appropriate diagnostic tools that can be used among culturally and linguistically diverse (CLD) children.
- Discuss general intervention principles for CLD children.
- Describe different service-delivery models provided to CLD children.

The American cultural landscape has been changing substantially, with an increase in various ethnic, racial, and linguistically diverse populations. Given the increase in diversity in the United States, there has been a compelling need to educate speech-language pathologists (SLPs) to recognize cultural and linguistic differences and their effect on clinical service. As the face of the United States changes, more professionals will need to operate in multicultural contexts, working with **culturally and linguistically diverse (CLD) populations**. For instance, the increase in diversity in the United States is reflected in many schools. The U.S. Census of 2000 reported that one in five school-aged children was a nonnative English speaker.

The American Speech-Language-Hearing Association (ASHA) has been recognizing the importance of multicultural issues and its effect on service delivery and has been developing policies and standards to provide guidance for SLPs working with CLD clients. Most recently, ASHA incorporated multicultural competencies within the content knowledge and skills standards required for certifying SLPs (ASHA, 2005). For instance, Standard III-C states: "The applicant must demonstrate knowledge of the nature of speech, language, hearing, and communication disorders and differences and swallowing disorders, including the etiologies, characteristics, anatomical/physiological, acoustic, psychological, developmental, and linguistic and cultural correlates" (ASHA, 2005).

Unfortunately, many SLPs and other school professionals who work with CLD children lack adequate training to provide these students with culturally and linguistically appropriate instruction and intervention (Eschevarria, Short, & Powers, 2006; Rosa-Lugo & Fradd, 2000; Roseberry-McKibbin & O'Hanlon, 2005). The lack of training among such professionals has led to the overrepresentation of CLD students in special education.

Changes in the cultural landscape of the United States and the unfortunate overrepresentation of CLD students in special education motivated the reauthorization of the original Individuals with Disabilities Education Improvement Act (IDEA 1997). The IDEA 2004 incorporated specific mandates regarding the assessment of CLD students, requiring school professionals to provide all students with linguistically and culturally appropriate assessment and instruction.

Professionals who are unaware of or disregard the effect of cultural influences on children's communication behaviors and language development may inadvertently contribute to the overrepresentation of CLD students in special education, which is not only unethical but also violates legal mandates.

Culture and Culturally and Linguistically Diverse Populations

As described by Battle (2002), **culture** "is about the behaviors, beliefs, and values of a group of people who are brought together by their commonality" (Battle, 2002, p. 3). According to Vecoli (1995), culture influences the way one perceives and interprets the world. An important aspect of a social cultural group is that their members share an underlying system of knowledge that allows them to know how to communicate with one another. As Battle pointed out (2002), one cannot understand communication by a group of individuals without an understanding of the cultural factors related to communication interactions in that group.

Culturally and linguistically diverse population is usually used to designate those who differ culturally and/or linguistically from Anglo-European mainstream Americans. To provide culturally and linguistically appropriate services, SLPs need to understand basic cultural characteristics that can potentially affect service delivery to a multicultural population. For instance, communication patterns can differ from culture to culture. SLPs not familiar with the communication patterns in the Native American community may misinterpret a Native American child's silence in one-to-one interaction with an adult as a communication disorder, when in reality it reflects a communication pattern in that cultural group.

As an instructor of speech-language pathology who teaches a course in multicultural issues in speech-language pathology, I like to share with my students my own experiences as an immigrant to this country and as a nonnative speaker of English. One of my favorite examples is my first visit to an American supermarket. I use this example to demonstrate to my students how language and communication are embedded in culture.

When I first came to the United States more than 10 years ago, I had limited proficiency in English. When I planned my first trip to the supermarket, I decided to take with me a 100-dollar bill so I would not have problems trying to figure out how much I had to pay for my groceries. At that time, I preferred to figure out whether the change that the cashier would give me was correct than to repeatedly ask the cashier how much I owed for my groceries. That was a common strategy among my Brazilian friends who, like me, had a limited knowledge of English. After the cashier scanned my grocery items, she inquired, "Paper or plastic?" Although I understood the words *paper* and *plastic*, I had no idea what she meant. After 10 seconds passed, which seemed more like 10 minutes, I replied, "What?" The cashier repeated in a louder voice to no avail, "Paper or plastic?" Again I understood the words, but I still had no clue what she meant. Five seconds more passed when I finally gave up and used one of my most reliable sentences, "I am sorry, but I don't speak English." The cashier promptly grabbed a paper bag and plastic bag and in an even louder voice said, "Do want paper or plastic?" as she waved the paper bag and plastic bag in front of me in slow motion.

For the people in line witnessing my communication exchange with the cashier, it might have appeared that I had experienced a language barrier due to my limited English proficiency, as validated by the statement,

"I don't speak English." However, cultural differences were also underlying that breakdown in communication. I definitely knew the meaning of the words paper and plastic, but in my home country, customers were never offered the option between paper and plastic bags while grocery shopping.

American English and Its Dialects

American English (AE) is commonly used to refer to the type of English used in the United States. As with other languages, AE includes a number of different **dialects**, among which are mainstream American English (MAE, also referred as standard American English), African American English (AAE), and Appalachian English. Dialect can be defined as any variety of a language used by a group of individuals that reflects and is determined by shared social, cultural/ethnic, and regional factors (Wolfram, 1991). Dialects represent a legitimate rule-governed language system across all linguistic parameters (i.e., phonology, morphology, syntax, semantics, pragmatics). Although each AE dialect has distinguishing characteristics, all share basic common features to all varieties of AE. Indeed, there are at least 10 regional dialects in the United States (Owens, 2005), and, for the most part, Americans from different regions are still able to understand one another.

Although controversy surrounds the term MAE as reflecting a language prestige rather than a linguistic entity (Haynes, Moran, & Pindzola, 2006), it is usually used to refer to a variety of English representative of mainstream America, and the variety typically used by government, mass media, businesses, schools, and academic settings in the United States. According to ASHA, all dialects represent a functional and effective variety of American English, and, therefore, it is the ASHA's position that no dialectal variety of AE should be considered a speech or language disorder (ASHA, 2003).

Language Differences Versus Language-Learning Disability

SLPs need to consider cultural and linguistic differences to select appropriate assessment tools, to make accurate judgments about the existence of a disorder, and to set treatment goals. Many cultural groups living in the United States will exhibit differences in their communication and language that reflect bilingual/bidialectal influences on English.

Although such influence can be present in any area of communication, language seems to be significantly affected by such differences.

To understand and recognize such influence, clinicians need to develop some degree of cultural competence, that is, to be aware of and acquire knowledge about different cultural groups. When working with CLD children, SLPs need to understand and recognize sociocultural influences on language development and acquisition. This is particularly important when trying to differentiate between **language differences** and **language-learning disability (LLD)**. To make an accurate assessment of language disabilities among CLD children, SLPs have to try to answer the following question: Do the child's linguistic variations reflect regular patterns in the child's dialect/primary language (language differences) or represent true language-learning disabilities? If the child's speech and language variations reflect dialect/primary language rules, such variations do not indicate a speech or language disorder.

SLPs need to have a basic understanding of how different dialects and languages influence the production of MAE (Roseberry-McKibbin, 2008) and how their culture influences the way they communicate with others. For instance, it is very common for children who are learning a second language to transfer the characteristics of their primary language (the language the child learned first and used most frequently in the early stages of language development) to the other language. This phenomenon is known as **language transference** (interference). Language differences in sentence structure, pronunciation, vocabulary, and pragmatics are frequently observed among second-language learners, and many times are the consequence of a transference process (Swan & Smith, 2004). Such differences usually reflect the child's primary language/dialect's morphology, syntax, semantics, pragmatics, and phonology, which are transferred to the second language, especially in the early stages of the second-language acquisition.

The language pattern from a primary language can definitely interfere with the way one phrases a particular message in a second language. For instance, my daughter (a Portuguese-English speaker) demonstrated some transference processes while learning English. When she was 3 years old, any time somebody would ask her how old she was in English, she would answer, "I have 3 years." In Brazilian Portuguese, "*Eu tenho tres anos*" means "I am 3 years old," but the literal translation in Portuguese would be "I have 3 years." Such transference can be misleading to novice SLPs or SLPs who do not have much experience working with CLD children. They can take differences from the mainstream English as a sign

Table 8–1 Examples of English Characteristics Observed Among AAE, Spanish, Asian, and Arabic Speakers

Languages	Articulatory and Phonological Characteristics	English Patterns and Utterances
AAE	Consonant cluster reduction	rus/rust
	Deletion of final consonant	hoo/hood
Spanish	*b/v* substitutions	bary/vary
	d or z /voiced *th*	dis/this, zat/that
Asian	*v/w* substitutions	vall/wall
	r/l confusion	croud/cloud
Arabic	*n/ng* substitutions	sin/sing
	Sch/ch substitutions	mush/much

Languages	Morphological and Syntactic Characteristics	English Patterns and Utterances
AAE	Omission of third person singular present tense marker	She like milk
	Present tense forms of auxiliary *have* are omitted	He been here before
Spanish	Past tense -ed is often omitted	We work yesterday
	Double negatives are used	I don't have no money
Asian	Omission of copula	She tired
	Omission of possessive	Dad drink is hot
Arabic	Omission of preposition	Put your clothes
	Inversion of noun constructs	Let's go to the station gas

Source: Adapted from Roseberry-McKibbin, 2008.

of language disability, which leads to incorrect diagnosis and erroneous placement of a child in special education.

With second-language learning, the more a learner is exposed to the second language and has experience in using the second language, the less likely language transference occurs. With that in mind, whenever an SLP is evaluating an **English-language learner (ELL)** child, she or he should consider the possibility that the "errors" may result from language transference or the child's lack of exposure and experience in using English. See **Table 8–1** for more examples of common transference processes among speakers of different languages in the United States.

Similarly, an understanding of dialectal characteristics is imperative for SLPs to avoid erroneous and unethical diagnosis when working with CLD children from various cultural groups in the United States (e.g., African American, Native American, Hispanic, and Asian) who speak a different dialect from the MAE. SLPs need to be able to differentiate which aspects of a child's speech and language reflect their dialectal patterns and which aspects indicate a disorder. For instance, when comparing MAE to AAE, children who speak AAE usually present as a dialectal pattern the *f/* voiceless *th* substitution at the end of words (e.g., *teef* for *teeth*; *bof* for *both*). See Table 8–1 for more examples of linguistic variations produced by AAE speakers. Good comprehensive resource books are available for SLPs to learn about linguistic variations among various cultural groups in the United States (e.g., Goldstein, 2000; Roseberry-McKibbin, 2008).

Heterogeneity Within Cultural Groups

SLPs need to keep in mind that, although cultural tendencies and linguistic patterns can be observed among various cultural groups, they need to recognize that not all members of a cultural group have the same values, beliefs, or customs. Part of being a culturally competent professional is to avoid overgeneralizations and stereotypes. There is a great heterogeneity within cultural groups. Many variables can influence the behavior and views of individuals within a culture, such as the person's age, gender, educational background (oneself and of family members), religious beliefs, length of residence in the country, degree of acculturation, languages spoken, generation membership, immigration status, and socioeconomic status (Battle, 2002; Roseberry-McKibbin, 2008).

Considering the heterogeneity within cultural groups, it is important to view a child as an individual first and foremost. Indeed, the interaction between general cultural practices and individual characteristics influences service delivery to CLD clients and their families (Battle, 2002). Another important aspect that SLPs need to consider is that even within each language group, there can also be great diversity. For instance, Spanish is a language spoken in different countries (Spain, all of Central America, and most counties of South America). Spanish speakers in the United States may speak different dialects or varieties of Spanish, depending on their background and origins (Mattes & García-Easterly, 2007; Mattes & Saldaña-Illingworth, 2008). Such heterogeneity can also be found among African Americans. Not all African Americans speak AAE, and like other dialects, its use may be influenced by geographical region, socioeconomic status, gender, education, and age (Craig, Washington, & Thompson-Porter, 1998; Long, 2006; Wyatt, 1998).

Processes of Second Language Acquisition and Bilingual Development

When professionals are assessing bilingual children's linguistic, cognitive, or academic skills, they need to understand and take into account the processes of second-language acquisition and bilingual development. Failure to consider such processes can preclude SLPs to distinguish accurately between language differences and language-learning disability (Gonzales, 2007; Restrepo & Kruth, 2000). Besides language transference, there are some other typical behaviors involved in bilingual development.

Code Switching (Code Mixing)

Code switching is a natural component of **bilingualism** and refers to a speaker's use of a word, phrase, or sentence from one language/dialect when communicating in the other language/dialect. Such alternation between two languages is common among bilingual communities, which is used by proficient bilinguals, not only in the United States but all over the world (Centeno, 2007; Genesee, Paradis, & Crago, 2004). It can serve social and pragmatic purposes when a speaker is communicating in two languages or two dialects (Seymour & Roeper, 1999). Some contextual situations are particularly conducive to code switching, such as the need to emphasize the group identity, show expertise, and quote someone (Grosjean, 1982). Another contextual situation that is conducive of code switching is when a speaker uses a word or phrase that may not have an equivalent in the other language. For instance, in Brazilian Portuguese, the word *saudade* can be described as an emptiness when referring to something or someone that should be there in a particular moment but is missing, and the person feels this absence. There is not an equivalent word in English. It is very common among Brazilians living in the United States to incorporate in their discourse the word *saudade*, especially when relating their feelings of homesickness.

Code switching is a common communicative behavior among children learning a second language (Genesee et al., 2004). During the early stages of a second-language acquisition, children may use code switching as a strategy to substitute structures, forms, or lexical items from the primary language into the second language that has not yet been learned. The frequency of code switching among bilingual children also varies, with the context of interaction being one important variable (Oller, Oller, & Badon, 2006). Although code switching is a natural component of bilingualism, its excessive presence may indicate a person's lack of proficiency in one of the languages.

Silent Period

Some second-language learners can go through what is known as a **silent period** in which there is little verbal output and much listening and comprehension (Brice, 2002). It seems that, during such a period, second-language learners are concentrating on learning the rules of the second language and are many times covertly rehearsing what they are learning (Hegde & Maul, 2006). Although the length of a silent period may vary from learner to learner (Paradis, 2007), lasting anywhere from 3 to 6 months, generally the younger the child is when exposed to the second language, the longer the silent period lasts (Tabors, 1997). Not aware of such a silent period, SLPs might misinterpret it as a sign of expressive language delay.

Language Loss

Unfortunately, it is common for second-language learners to lose their first language, if its use is decreased (Anderson, 2004; Brice, 2002; Mattes & García-Easterly, 2007). Such **language loss** process has been observed as a shift in proficiency with second-language learners losing skills in the first language, as proficiency is acquired in the second language. Different factors have been associated with language loss among bilingual communities (Anderson, 2004); however, an important factor is the lack of opportunity for exposure and experience in using the first language. This is particularly the case among children who attend schools where bilingual education is not offered, with the children hearing and speaking only the second language in the academic environment. Frequently, the maintenance of a primary language is often the result of families' efforts to maintain its use at home (Langdon, 2008).

Many CLD children in the United States tend to lose their first language, as their first language is gradually replaced by English (Gonzales, 2007; Paradis, 2007). This process may be particularly misleading when a second-language learner loses his or her skills in the primary language while he or she is still acquiring language skills in a second language. The lack of skills in both languages may be erroneously considered symptomatic of a language disability and poses increasing challenges for the SLP to differentiate between language differences and language-learning disabilities.

Common Misconceptions About Bilingualism

Parents and even some SLPs often assume that bilingualism causes language-learning disability. Although some SLPs and parents might have this misconception, bilingualism does not cause LLD. Bilingual children with LLD will have difficulties learning any language (Roseberry & Connell, 1991). The simultaneous exposure to and use of more than one language is not harmful for the child and does not represent a too-demanding cognitive task for the child if the language-learning environment provides adequate support for the development of those languages (Genesee, 2003). Studies demonstrate that bilingual children show no difference in their performance on phonologic, syntactic, or lexical tasks as compared with monolingual children (Bosh & Sebastian-Gallés, 2001; Umbel & Oller, 1994). Bilingualism, however, can be advantageous for children. Studies show that bilingualism seems to have positive effects on different measures of linguistic and cognitive development. The most frequently reported findings indicate that bilingual children exhibit advanced metalinguistic skills relative to monolingual counterparts (Bialystok, 2001).

Besides cognitive and linguistic benefits, bilingualism can also bring some economic advantages. In the current globalized economy, bilinguals may have advantages in the job market. Another important aspect of bilingualism is that, for many bilingual children, maintaining a primary language is the only or main way to communicate with family members or members of their cultural background.

Language Differences and Language-Learning Disability Among English-Language Learner Children

Many SLPs struggle when trying to distinguish language differences from a language-learning disability (Oller et al., 2006; Roseberry-McKibbin & O'Hanlon, 2005). This can be even more problematic when assessing bilingual populations. A good rule of thumb for SLPs to consider when assessing ELL children is that, if a child has a real language-learning disability, such a disability would underlie the child's ability to learn any language, including the child's primary language (Mattes & García-Easterly, 2007; Roseberry-McKibbin, 2008). In other words, to diagnose a language-learning disability appropriately, communication problems have to be evident in both English and the primary language.

Unfortunately, ELL children who are struggling in school are frequently referred to special education when in reality they may lack sufficient exposure to or experience using English in different contexts. An important aspect of language acquisition is language exposure and experience. The more exposure and experience in using a language, the more likely the learner will become competent in that language and most likely fewer language differences will be observed. SLPs need to take into account the child's degree of exposure and opportunities while learning English to make an accurate diagnosis. A second-language learner may not be learning because of lack of exposure to the language and lack of experience in using it. Professionals working with bilingual children need to consider the type of bilingualism and the proficiency level in each language, as well as the contexts in which the languages have been used. Taking into account the level of a child's exposure and experience in using a second language is important not only for diagnosis purposes but also for decisions regarding intervention.

Social and Academic Language Proficiencies

Professionals who work with ELL children must differentiate between social and academic language proficiencies. They must also be aware of their development timeline. Cummins's model of communicative proficiency (Cummins, 1984) clearly differentiates between language proficiency involved in context-embedded social interactions, which is referred to as **basic interpersonal communication skills (BICS)**, and language proficiency involved in context-reduced academic settings, which is referred to as **cognitive academic language proficiency (CALP)**. While it takes the average second-language learner 2 years under ideal conditions to develop BICS (Cummins, 1992), it may take 5 to 7 years for a second-language learner to develop CALP to a level commensurate with that of a native speaker (Cummins, Chow, & Schecter, 2006; Torres-Guzman, 2002).

Researchers have been pointing out that these timelines can even be longer, with low-income second-language learners often taking more than 2 years to develop BICS (Hakuta, Butler, & Witt, 2000). Some second-language learners have been reported to take between 7 and 10 years to develop native-like level of CALP under less than optimal exposure conditions to the second language (Eschevarria et al., 2006).

Language proficiency tests are generally given to assess schoolchildren's level of proficiency in English. However, these tests seem to assess only BICS. Although ELL children who take these proficiency tests might receive a label of "fully proficient," in reality, their CALP skills were not assessed (Roseberry-McKibbin, 2008). With such a label, professionals are sought to be given a green light to administer monolingual, norm-referenced tests and academic measures to these children, which in general leads to low scores. The potential BICS–CALP gap may mislead professionals to conclude that ELL children have a language-learning disability and need special education assessment and intervention (Chamberlain, 2005).

Response to Intervention Approach

A response to intervention (RtI) approach has been described as an important prereferral intervention that can help teachers to assess appropriately the needs of their students and the possible need for a special education evaluation (Chamberlain, 2005). RtI may be used as a form of dynamic assessment to evaluate children's ability to learn when provided with appropriate instruction. When CLD children do not respond appropriately to a well-planned RtI, while their peers with similar cultural and linguistic backgrounds respond to it, it may indicate an appropriate referral for a special education evaluation (Chamberlain, 2005; Ortiz, 2001). RtI was mandated in the IDEA (2004) as a way to avoid overreferral of certain groups of students to special education. Indeed, ASHA (2007) stated that a child's response to RtI should be used for educational decisions, including the child's inclusion in an SLP's caseload. Children who do not respond well to RtI should be referred for a comprehensive speech-language evaluation.

Assessing CLD children

Although there is not a specific procedure to assess CLD children, many experts in the field have been suggesting a need for using multiple assessment measures (Roseberry-McKibbin, 2008; Stockman, 1996). SLPs need to assess CLD children across a variety of tasks and contexts, and, ideally for bilingual children, in both languages.

For those cases in which an overall assessment of language abilities is necessary, informal procedures should supplement the results of standardized tests. Indeed, the administration of a single standardized test does not usually provide an SLP with sufficient information for a differential diagnosis, and this is especially true when the SLP is evaluating CLD children. In fact, standardized tests can pose many difficulties, especially when they are used among CLD populations.

When selecting standardized tests, SLPs must remember that test norms are not valid or meaningful if the norming sample differs significantly from the tested population. This is an essential psychometric rule that is true for any type of population being assessed, multicultural or not. Most standardized tests in English are normed in MAE and are highly biased against CLD children and therefore not appropriate measures of performance for many of those children (Roseberry-McKibbin & O'Hanlon, 2005).

Although some efforts have been made to incorporate multicultural groups in the norming samples of standardized tests, the percentage of these children may not represent the proportion of such groups in local areas, as pointed out by Haynes and Pindzola (2008). In addition, given the heterogeneity among cultural groups, unless specific information about the multicultural groups is provided (i.e., socioeconomic status, bidialectal/bilingual status) such representation might not be meaningful for the target population being tested.

Even tests developed in a primary language can also be biased. Spanish-speaking children can be given a Spanish test; however, given the heterogeneity among populations who speak Spanish, the standardization norm can be misleading. For instance, some words frequently used by Spanish speakers in one area of the United States may be rarely used in other parts of the country (Mattes & García-Easterly, 2007).

Besides linguistic biases, there are also cultural biases associated with standardized tests (Figueroa & Newsome, 2006; Oller et al., 2006). In my experience taking the graduate record examinations for graduate school many years ago, I was unable to answer a question that required knowledge about the shape of a baseball field. Although I knew the algebra necessary to answer the question, I had no idea of the shape of a baseball field. At that time, baseball was not played in my home country. Any task or items that do not make part of the child's repertoire of experiences have the potential for biases.

Many SLPs use translated versions of English tests when working with CLD clients. Translated tests can have inherent linguistic and cultural biases (Carter et al., 2005; Mattes & Saldaña-Illingworth, 2008). Direct translation of tests do not account for differences in background/life experiences. In addition, structural and content characteristics inherent to a primary language may not have a correspondent component to English. For instance, in Brazilian Portuguese, like in Spanish, words for the article *the* vary, depending on whether the following noun is masculine (e.g., *o garoto* = the boy), feminine (e.g., *a garota* = the girl), singular (*o carro* = the car), or plural (*os carros* = the cars). Direct translation from tests in English would not address the definite article variations in Portuguese.

Different ways to alter the administration and interpretation of standardized tests have also been proposed to diminish the biases against CLD children (Carter et al., 2005; Wilson, Wilson, & Coleman, 2000). The main goal of such alterations is to allow for a more accurate picture of children's true ability and may include giving extra time for a child to respond and, if necessary, allocating more than one session to the testing; providing instructions in both English and the primary language; repeating items whenever necessary; and skipping biased items. Another alteration that can be considered is computing more than one score (dual scoring system). The SLP can compute one score that reflects the procedures used with the normative sample and another score reflecting possible cultural/linguistic adjustments, including also items answered in the child's primary language/dialect.

Although such alternative scoring systems are helpful in diminishing biases against CLD children, they are far from a definitive solution to the use of standardized tests among ELL children or children who speak a dialect other than MAE. Norms still cannot be used because the test was not scored the same way as it was during the test development. SLPs have to keep in mind that any time departures from standard testing procedures occur, they have to be clearly reported in the assessment report, with detailed cautions and disclaimers.

For the past 30 years, many standardized tests have been developed in other languages, especially Spanish. However, very few have been properly normed on monolingual or bilingual populations. The *Clinical Evaluation of Language Fundamentals* (CELF-4) (Semel, Wiig, & Secord, 2005) was normed in bilingual Spanish-speaking students residing in different regions of the United States, with approximately 30 percent of them living in households in which English was spoken more than 96 percent of the time.

There has also been a recent effort in the development of more culturally fair and dialectally nonbiased standardized language tests for children who are speakers of dialects other than the MAE. *The Diagnostic*

Evaluation of Language Variation (DELV) is available in three editions: The screening edition (Seymour, Roeper, De Villiers, & De Villiers 2003a), the criterion-referenced edition (Seymour, Roeper, De Villiers, & De Villiers, 2003b), and the norm-referenced edition (Seymour, Roeper, De Villiers, & De Villiers, 2005). The DELV can be used for the language assessment of all children (aged 4 through 9 years), including those children who are speakers of dialects other than MAE. The DELV assesses a variety of language parameters (syntax, phonology, semantics, and pragmatics) and yields important information for differentiating language differences from language disorders. Preliminary studies have been showing that this test is sensitive to the linguistic and cultural differences represented by many African American children as a valid tool for differentiating between language differences and language disorders, as well as identifying children at risk for a language impairment (Seymour, Roeper, & De Villiers, 2004).

Because of the problems generally associated with standardized tests, many experts in the field have been recommending using informal procedures, either alone or in conjunction with standardized tests, for assessing CLD children's language skills (Gonzales, 2007; McLaughlin, 2006; Roseberry-McKibbin, 2008). Among such informal assessments are the following:

1. *Dynamic assessment*: A child is evaluated over time in a test-teach-retest format. This assessment approach focuses on the child's capacity to learn rather than exclusively focusing on what the child already knows or does not know (Peña et al., 2006; Peña, Iglesias, & Lidz, 2001). The assumption behind using **dynamic assessment** in dealing with CLD children is that children who can learn language in a short period when appropriate instruction is provided probably have normal language-learning abilities. However, children who still have difficulties learning linguistic-based materials, even though appropriate stimulation is provided during a dynamic assessment, may be more likely to demonstrate language-learning difficulties.

2. *Multiple observations in naturalistic settings*: SLPs should observe the child's communication skills in different, everyday contexts (e.g., in the classroom, at recess, at lunch, and at home)

3. *Language samples*: Collect language samples in different sociocultural contexts to evaluate the child's communication skills. In the case of bilingual children, the samples should be collected ideally in both languages.

4. *Informal comparison*: Comparing a second-language learner to a child with a similar language background can provide important information for the assessment of an ELL child (Langdon, 2008). Indeed, among possible indicators of a language-learning disability is the parents' report of a child's slower development as compared with siblings.

5. *Interview*: Obtain an accurate and detailed history of the child's primary language development. This is even more important if assessment in that language is not possible because of lack of personnel fluent in the child's primary language or because of lack of appropriate assessment tools (Langdon, 2008). When interviewing parents, SLPs should be particularly attentive to reports of communication difficulties at home, family history of special education and learning difficulties, child's reliance on gestures rather than speech to communicate, and difficulty learning language at a normal rate, even with special assistance in both languages. In addition, it is important to collect information about the child's level of experience in the primary language, including information about his or her literacy experience in the primary language.

6. *Questionnaires*: SLPs can use questionnaires to obtain information about the child's communicative functioning in daily contexts from people who interact with the child.

Intervention for CLD Children

As discussed before, when considering speech-language disorders, children need to exhibit difficulties that affect performance in all languages/dialects they speak to be included in an SLP's caseload. If children's language difficulties reflect a second-language acquisition pattern or dialectal differences rather than a disability, these children should not receive special education services. In the case of bilingual children who are struggling in school, if they do not qualify for special education, they should receive services from other school resource personnel including classroom teachers, English as a second language (ESL) teachers, bilingual personnel, tutors, etc.

Service-Delivery Models

There is a range of services available for CLD children, once comprehensive assessment determines that they qualify for special education (Roseberry-McKibbin, 2008). The availability of each service varies from school to school and many times depends on school personnel and individual states' policies and laws. Such services may include the following:

1. Pull-out services: The child goes to the specialist's room once or twice a week for individual or small-group intervention in English (or hopefully bilingual intervention).
2. Consultative/collaborative services: The child continues in a regular classroom and the teacher receives assistance from special education personnel, an ESL teacher, and/or bilingual staff.
3. Placement in a regular bilingual classroom with support from special education.
4. Placement in a bilingual special education classroom.
5. Placement in a monolingual English special education classroom, hopefully with primary language support through a bilingual teacher, tutor, or others.

SLPs are being highly encouraged to shift from a traditional intervention approach (e.g., individual pull-out once or twice a week) to a more classroom-based intervention approach, where more time is spent in the classroom in collaboration with the teachers (Nelson, 2007). SLPs collaborate with teachers to help children to succeed in the academic and social setting of the classroom.

General Intervention Principles

When planning an intervention program for CLD children who qualify for special education services, SLPs need to do the following:

1. Focus on language skills the children need to be successful in the school setting. The focus should be in activities that support classroom curriculum and help children learn classroom content.
2. Focus on activities that promote CLD children's effective interaction with their classmates.
3. Focus on meaning, rather than on structure. To be effective, intervention should promote learning of concepts and strategies in authentic communication situations (Brice, 2002; Oller et al., 2006).
4. Consider the unique characteristics of the child. To facilitate learning, the SLP should use activities that are culturally meaningful to the child.
5. Work collaboratively with the child's parents while developing treatment goals. The SLP must take into account the parents' input to avoid cultural conflicts and misunderstanding while setting goals.

Intervention Issues for Bilingual Children

SLPs need to be particularly cautioned when planning an intervention for potential phonologic disorders among CLD children. If a CLD child has a problem pronouncing a particular sound or sound combination, the SLP needs to make sure that the pattern is actually deviant and not a reflection of language/dialectal differences. If the SLP is not familiar with the child's primary language, she or he needs to gather information about the language and possible transference processes (possible resources: books, members of the community who speak the child's primary language, linguistic departments at universities, etc.). In addition, parents and other individuals who know the child may be a valuable source of information as far as identifying or reporting phonologic difficulties when the child is communicating in the primary language.

Language Choice for Intervention

There is no coherent literature addressing language choice for intervention (Kohnert, 2004) that can direct SLPs to one direction or the other. However, ideally, intervention should take place in both languages (Goldstein, 2004). Treatment in both languages is recommended because, although gains in one language can also promote gains in the other language, not all remediated processes transfer from one language to the other. For instance, Holm, Dodd, and Ozonne (1997) reported that an intervention provided in English for a Japanese–English-speaking child successfully enabled the child to pronounce s in both languages but not consonant clusters. Whereas the child was able to pronounce clusters in English, the intervention fell short when it came time to transfer the ability to Japanese, most likely because of specific phonologic differences between the languages.

Many SLPs often recommend that parents of bilingual children with cognitive and language disorders restrict speaking to their children in just one language (Thordardottir, 2006). They believe that bilingual exposure can be detrimental to those children. However, current studies show that exposure to a bilingual environment is not detrimental for children with language and cognitive impairments. For instance, Kay-Raining Bird et al. (2005) reported comparable English-language progress between children with Down syndrome growing up in a bilingual environment and a matched group of monolingual English-speaking children with Down syndrome. In their study, the children growing up in a bilingual environment performed as well as their monolingual counterparts on different English tasks. Paradis, Crago, Genesee, and Rice (2003) reported that

French–English bilingual children with language impairments exhibited the same type and frequency of morphosyntactic errors as monolingual French and English controls subject with language impairments.

Negative consequences for children and their families can result from limiting language input to a single language. For instance, such limitation can isolate children from important cultural contexts shared with other family members. Limiting language input to a single language might also affect parent–child natural interaction, if parents (many times following the SLP recommendation) select a language that they are not very comfortable speaking.

Family support is important when SLPs are working with CLD children who exhibit language-learning difficulties (Langdon, 2008). With bilingual children, parents need to be reassured that speaking the primary language at home is not detrimental to their children's linguistic and educational progress and that they, too, are teachers of their children. Indeed, family members, as well as members of the child's cultural community, are important to promoting intervention success by helping the children to expand the variety of uses for the primary language.

Speech-Language Pathologists' Bilingual Status

As mentioned earlier, ideally, intervention should take place in both languages and, therefore, should be conducted by an SLP who is bilingual and fluent in the child's primary language. If a bilingual SLP is not available, an alternative would be for the SLP to work collaboratively with an interpreter or bilingual paraprofessionals (Kohnert, Yim, Nett, Kan, & Duran, 2005). When such professionals are unavailable, the SLP ends up conducting the intervention entirely in English. The latter intervention scenario is the most common because of the limited number of bilingual SLPs in the United States and the lack of bilingual personnel in schools. When the SLP is unable to provide bilingual intervention to the child and no bilingual staff is available for collaboration, the SLP must emphasize the importance of maintaining the primary language at home. Parents and family members can have an active role in the intervention process by facilitating the primary language development at home.

Other Factors Related to Language Choice for Intervention

1. *The primary language reflects the cultural environment in which the child is raised*: The primary language continues to be the

dominant language for most aspects of the child's communication in the home environment and therefore needs to be maintained.

2. *Potential language loss*: It can jeopardize the child's ability to communicate with family members who speak only the primary language (Mattes & Garcia-Easterly, 2007). Studies show that parents and children who interact in the primary language report a more close and emotionally authentic relationship (Tannenbaum, 2005; Yan, 2003), and primary language loss can be detrimental to the quality of the parent–child relationship in those cases where parents speak little or no English (Cummins, 2000).

3. *Child's language preference*: It is important to consider the child's language preference and his or her attitudes about the primary language and motivation to maintain it.

4. *Parents' language preference*: Some parents are vehement in maintaining the primary language and feel that intervention should be provided in both languages. Other parents, wishing to speed up the child's English development, may prefer English-only intervention. SLPs should educate these parents regarding the advantages of bilingualism and the importance of maintaining and developing the child's primary language, so that they can make more conscious decisions while provided with adequate information about the subject.

Chapter Summary

This chapter provides a framework for SLPs to develop an understanding of the many issues related to assessment and intervention for children from various cultural and linguistic backgrounds. The importance of differentiating between language differences and language-learning disability is highlighted in this chapter, with a description of typical behaviors associated with bilingual development and cultural differences that affect children's communication behaviors. Different diagnostic tools for CLD children are discussed in this chapter to help SLPs to make an appropriate diagnosis and to avoid overrepresentation of CLD children in special education. Finally, the importance of bilingualism and bilingual intervention is highlighted in this chapter.

MULTICULTURAL ISSUES IN ASSESSMENT AND INTERVENTION

Terms from the Chapter

American English *(128)*
Basic interpersonal communication
  skills *(135)*
Bilingualism *(132)*
Code switching *(132)*
Cognitive academic language
  proficiency *(135)*
Culturally and linguistically
  diverse (CLD) populations *(125)*
Culture *(126)*

Dialects *(128)*
Dynamic assessment *(139)*
English-language learner *(130)*
Language differences *(129)*
Language-learning disability *(129)*
Language loss *(133)*
Language transference *(129)*
Response to intervention
  approach *(136)*
Silent period *(133)*

References

American Speech-Language-Hearing Association. (2003). *American English dialects* [Technical Report]. Retrieved from www.asha.org/policy

American Speech-Language-Hearing Association. (2005). *2005 standards and implementation procedures for the certificate of clinical competence in speech-language pathology.* Retrieved from http://www.asha.org/certification/slp_standards.htm#Std_III

American Speech-Language-Hearing Association. (2007). Responsiveness to intervention (RtI). Retrieved from http://www.asha.org/members/slp/schools/prof-consult/RtI.htm

Anderson, R. (2004). Children: Patterns of loss and implications for clinical practice. Influences, contexts, and processes. In B. A. Goldstein (Ed.), *Bilingual language development and disorders in Spanish-English speakers* (pp. 187–211). Baltimore, MD: Paul H. Brookes.

Battle, D. E. (2002). Communication disorders in a multicultural society. In D. Battle (Ed.), *Communication disorders in multicultural populations* (3rd ed., pp. 33–70). Stoneham, MA: Butterworth-Heinemann.

Bialystok, E. (2001). *Bilingualism in development: Language, literacy, and cognition.* New York: Cambridge University Press.

Bosh, L., & Sebastián-Gallés, N. (2001). Early language differentiation in bilingual infants. In J. Cenoz & F. Genesee (Eds.), *Trends in bilingual acquisition* (pp. 231–256). Amsterdam, The Netherlands: John Benjamins.

Brice, A. E. (2002). *The Hispanic child: Speech, language, culture, and education.* Boston, MA: Allyn & Bacon.

Carter, J. A., Lees, J. A., Murira, G. M., Gona, J., Neville, B. G. R., & Newton, C. R. J. C. (2005). Issues in the development of cross-cultural assessments of speech and language for children. *International Journal of Language & Communication Disorders, 40,* 385–401.

Centeno, J. G. (2007). From theory to realistic praxis: Service-learning as a teaching method to enhance speech-language services with minority populations. In A. J. Wurr & J. Hellenbrandt (Eds.), *Learning the language of global citizenship: Service-learning in applied linguistics* (pp. 190–218). Boston, MA: Anker Publishing.

Chamberlain, S. P. (2005). Recognizing and responding to cultural differences in the education of culturally and linguistically diverse learners. *Intervention in School and Clinic, 40,* 195–211.

Craig, H. K., Washington, J. A., & Thompson-Porter, C. (1998). Average C-unit lengths in the discourse of African American children from low-income, urban homes. *Journal of Speech-Language-Hearing Research, 41*(2), 433–444.

Cummins, J. (1984). *Bilingualism and special education.* Clevedon, UK: Multilingual Matters.

Cummins, J. (1992). The role of primary language development in promoting educational success for language minority students. In C. Leyba (Ed.), *Schooling and language minority students: A theoretical framework.* Los Angeles: California State University.

Cummins, J. (2000). *Language, power and pedagogy: Bilingual children in the cross-fire.* Clevedon, UK: Multilingual Matters.

Cummins, J., Chow, P., & Schecter, S. R. (2006). Community as curriculum. *Language Arts, 83,* 297–307.

Eschevarria, J., Short, D., & Powers, K. (2006). School reform and standards-based education: A model for English-language learners. *Journal of Educational Research, 99,* 195–211.

Figueroa, R. A., & Newsome, P. (2006). The diagnosis of learning disability in English learners. *Journal of Learning Disabilities, 39,* 206–214.

Genesee, F. (2003). Rethinking bilingual acquisition. In J. Dewaele, A. Housen, & L. Wei (Eds.), *Bilingualism: Beyond basic principles* (pp. 204–229). Clevedon, UK: Multilingual Matters.

Genesee, F., Paradis, J., & Crago, M. B. (2004). *Dual language development and disorders: A handbook on bilingualism and second language learners.* Baltimore, MD: Paul H. Brookes.

Goldstein, B. (2000). *Cultural and linguistic diversity resource guide for speech-language pathologists.* San Diego, CA: Singular Publishing.

Goldstein, B. A. (2004). Bilingual language development and disorders: Introduction and overview. In B. A. Goldstein (Ed.), *Bilingual language development and disorders in Spanish-English speakers* (pp. 3–20). Baltimore, MD: Paul H. Brookes.

Gonzales, D. (2007). *Evaluating bilingual students for eligibility as speech/language impaired: A handbook for evidence-based decision-making.* Houston, TX: Region 4 Education Service Center.

Grosjean, F. (1982). *Life with two languages*. Cambridge, MA: Harvard University Press.

Hakuta, K., Butler, Y. G., & Witt, D. (2000). *How long does it take English learners to attain proficiency?* Santa Barbara: University of California Linguistic Minority Research Institute.

Haynes, W., Moran, M., & Pindzola, R. (2006). *Communication disorders in the classroom: An introduction for professionals in school settings*. Sudbury, MA: Jones and Bartlett.

Haynes, W., & Pindzola, R. (2008). *Diagnosis and evaluation in speech pathology* (7th ed.). Pearson Education.

Hegde, M. N., & Maul, C. A. (2006). *Language disorders in children: An evidence-based approach to assessment and treatment*. Boston, MA: Allyn & Bacon.

Holm, A., Dodd, H., & Ozonne, A. (1997). Efficacy of intervention for a bilingual child making articulation and phonological errors. *International Journal of Bilingualism, 1*, 55–69.

Kay-Raining Bird, E., Cleave, P., Trudeau, N., Thordardottir, E., Sutton, A., & Thorpe, A. (2005). The language abilities of bilingual children with Down syndrome. *American Journal of Speech-Language Pathology, 14*, 187–199.

Kohnert, K. (2004). Processing skills in early sequential bilinguals. In B. A. Goldstein (Ed.), *Bilingual language development and disorders in Spanish-English speakers* (pp. 53–76). Baltimore, MD: Paul H. Brookes.

Kohnert, K., Yim, D., Nett, K., Kan, P. F., & Duran, L. (2005). Intervention with linguistically diverse preschool children: A focus on developing home languages. *Language, Speech, and Hearing Services in Schools, 36*, 251–264.

Langdon, H. W. (2008). *Assessment and intervention for communication disorders in culturally and linguistically diverse populations*. Clifton Park, NY: Delmar, Cengage Learning.

Long, S. H. (2006). Language and linguistically-culturally diverse children. In V. A. Reed (Ed.), *An introduction to children with language disorders* (3rd ed., pp. 301–334). Boston, MD: Allyn & Bacon.

Mattes, L. J., & García-Easterly, I. (2007). *Bilingual speech and language intervention resource*. Oceanside, CA: Academic Communication.

Mattes, L. J., & Saldaña-Illingworth, C. (2008). *Bilingual communication assessment resource: Tools for assessing speech, language, and learning*. Oceanside, CA: Academic Communication.

McLaughlin, S. (2006). *Introduction to language development* (2nd ed.). Clifton Park, NY: Thomson Delmar Learning.

Nelson, N. W. (2007). "Be-attitudes" for managing change in school-based practice. *ASHA Leader, 12*, 20–21.

Oller, J. W., Oller, S. D., & Badon, L. C. (2006). *Milestones: Normal speech and language development across the life span*. San Diego, CA: Plural Publishing.

Ortiz, A. A. (2001). English language learners with special needs: Effective instructional strategies. In O. Garcia & C. Baker (Eds.), *Bilingual education: An introductory reader* (pp. 281–285). Clevedon, UK: Multilingual Matters.

Owens, R. E. (2005). *Language development: An introduction* (6th ed.). Boston, MA: Allyn & Bacon.

Paradis, J. (2007). Second language acquisition in childhood. In E. Hoff & M. Shatz (Eds.), *Handbook of language development* (pp. 387–406). Oxford: Blackwell.

Paradis, J., Crago, M., Genesee, F., & Rice, M. (2003). French-English bilingual children with SLI: How do they compare with their monolingual peers? *Journal of Speech, Language, and Hearing Research, 46*, 113–127.

Peña, E. D., Gillam, R. B., Malek, M., Ruiz-Felter, R., Resendiz, M., Fiestas, C., & Sabel, T. (2006). Dynamic assessment of school-age children's narrative ability: An experimental investigation of classification accuracy. *Journal of Speech, Language, and Hearing Research, 49*, 1037–1057.

Peña, E. D., Iglesias, A., & Lidz, C. S. (2001). Reducing test bias through dynamic assessment of children's word learning ability. *American Journal of Speech-Language Pathology, 10*(2), 138–154.

Restrepo, M. A., & Kruth, K. (2000). Grammatical characteristics of Spanish-English child with specific language impairment. *Communication Disorders Quarterly, 21*, 66–76.

Rosa-Lugo, L. I., & Fradd, S. (2000). Preparing professionals to serve English-language learners with communication disorders. *Communication Disorders Quarterly, 22*, 29–42.

Roseberry, C., & Connell, P. J. (1991). The use of invented language rule in the differentiation of normal and language-impaired Spanish-speaking children. *Journal of Speech and Hearing Research, 34*, 596–603.

Roseberry-McKibbin, C. (2008). *Multicultural students with special language needs* (3rd ed.). Oceanside, CA: Academic Communication.

Roseberry-McKibbin, C., & O'Hanlon, L. (2005). Nonbiased assessment of English language learners: A tutorial. *Communication Disorders Quarterly, 26*, 178–185.

Semel, E., Wiig, E. H., & Secord, W. (2005). *Clinical evaluation of language fundamentals* [CELF-4] [Spanish]. San Antonio, TX: Psychological Corporation.

Seymour, H. N., & Roeper, T. W. (1999). Grammatical acquisition of African American English. In O. Taylor & L. Leonard (Eds.), *Language acquisition across North America: Cross-cultural and cross-linguistic perspectives* (pp. 109–152). San Diego, CA: Singular.

Seymour, H. N., Roeper, T. W., & De Villiers, J. (2004). *Diagnostic Evaluation of Language Variation*. San Antonio, TX : Psychological corporation.

Seymour, H. N., Roeper, T. W., De Villiers, J., & De Villiers, P. (2003a). *Diagnostic evaluation of language variation screening test* [DELV]. San Antonio, TX: Psychological Corporation.

Seymour, H. N., Roeper, T. W., De Villiers, J., & De Villiers, P. (2003b). *Diagnostic evaluation of language variation (DELV)—Criterion referenced.* San Antonio, TX: Psychological Corporation.

Seymour, H. N., Roeper, T. W., De Villiers, J., & De Villiers, P. (2005). *Diagnostic evaluation of language variation (DELV)—Norm referenced.* San Antonio, TX: Psychological Corporation.

Stockman, I. J. (1996). The promises and pitfalls of language sample analysis as an assessment tool for linguistic minority children. *Language, Speech, and Hearing Services in Schools, 27,* 355–366.

Swan, M., & Smith, B. (2004). *Learner English: A teacher's guide to interference and other problems.* Cambridge, England: Cambridge University Press.

Tabors, P. O. (1997). *One child, two languages.* Baltimore, MD: Paul H. Brookes.

Tannenbaum, M. (2005). Viewing family relations through a linguistic lens: Symbolic aspects of language maintenance in immigrant families. *Journal of Family Communication, 5,* 229–252.

Thordardottir, E. (2006, August 15). Language intervention from a bilingual mindset. *ASHA Leader, 11,* 6–7, 20–21.

Torres-Guzman, M. E. (2002). Dual language programs: Key features and results. In O. Garcia & C. Baker (Eds.), *Bilingual education: An introductory reader* (pp. 50–63). Clevedon, UK: Multilingual Matters.

Umbel, V., & Oller, K. (1994). Developmental changes in receptive vocabulary in Hispanic bilingual school children. *Language Learning, 44,* 221–242.

US Bureau of the Census. (2000). *Statistical abstract of the United States, 2000* (120th ed.). Washington, DC: U.S. Department of Commerce.

Vecoli, R. J. (1995). Introduction. In J. Galens, A. Sheets, & R. V. Young (Eds.), *Gale encyclopedia of multicultural America* (pp. 21–27). New York, NY: Gale Research.

Wilson, F., Wilson, J. R., & Coleman, T. J. (2000). Culturally appropriate assessment: Issues and strategies. In T. J. Coleman (Ed.), *Clinical management of communication disorders in culturally diverse children* (pp. 202–238). Needham Heights, MA: Allyn & Bacon.

Wolfram, W. (1991). *Dialects and American English.* Englewood Cliffs, NJ: Prentice Hall.

Wyatt, T. (1998). Children's language development. In C. M. Seymour & E. H. Nober (Eds.), *Introduction to communication disorders: A multicultural approach* (pp. 59–86). Newton, MA: Butterworth-Heinemann.

Yan, R. (2003). Parental perceptions on maintaining heritage languages of CLD students. *Bilingual Review, 27,* 99–113.

C H A P T E R   9

Evidence-Based Practice

Ronald B. Hoodin

Chapter Objectives

After reading this chapter, you should be able to:

- Define the concept of evidence-based practice (EBP).
- Discuss the hierarchy of treatment efficacy evidence.
- Discuss the clinician-directed approaches with regard to EBP.
- Discuss the client-centered approaches with regard to EBP.
- Discuss the hybrid approaches with regard to EBP.
- Define the concept of single subject design (SSD).
- Discuss the application of SSD to demonstrate treatment efficacy with an individual child.

Evidence-based practice (EBP) has its roots in evidence-based medicine (EBM). EBM refers to the integration of research evidence, clinical expertise, and patient values (Sackett, Straus, Richardson, Rosenberg, & Haynes, 2000). In medicine, as well as its subdisciplines, this approach has pervaded clinical practice and research. EBP has also been embraced by the American Speech-Language-Hearing Association (ASHA, 2004). Although ASHA has embraced EBP on an organizational level, the individual clinician can make a commitment to EBP on a personal level.

Evidence-Based Practice

EBP does not simply mean that the treatment procedures are supported in the treatment literature. It also refers to making the best possible decisions and judgments. Therefore, EBP cannot be reduced to a simple mechanistic process. Rather, it is a much broader notion that presumes that the clinician keeps abreast of the professional literature. One major reason for embracing EBP is that clinical decision making should be based on actual evidence rather than relying on expert opinion. EBP is applicable not only to treatment efficacy but also to other areas, such as evaluating diagnostic procedures. Applying EBP criteria may resolve controversial diagnostic categories, including developmental apraxia of speech, auditory processing disorders, and nonverbal learning disability (ASHA, 2004).

On a practical level, it would be virtually impossible to review every single article and book on child language disorders to select a treatment approach. The alternative is to read published reviews of the literature. In addition, various library databases, such as MEDLINE, ERIC, WorldCat, and PsychInfo, are available to focus the search on articles that closely relate to the issue. Clinicians should use general search engines such as Google with caution because they are not limited to peer-reviewed articles. The designation of **peer reviewed** indicates that the article has passed a rigorous review process that reduces the potential for misinformation. The review of the literature should be critical. That is, the clinician needs to differentiate findings based on the quality of the evidence presented.

To help clinicians undertake a critical review of the literature, Hegde and Maul (2006) developed a hierarchy of treatment efficacy evidence for EBP (**Table 9–1**). As indicated in Table 9–1, clinicians should avoid using treatments solely based on **expert opinion**. Evidence derived from **uncontrolled investigations** is not much better. It lacks credibility because improvements associated with the treatment cannot be attributed to the treatment. Conversely, evidence derived from **controlled investigations** permits gains to be attributed to the treatment, a critical element in EBP. When controlled studies are **directly replicated**, their findings are likely to generalize across subjects. Controlled studies, which have been **systematically replicated**, represent an even higher form of evidence. The findings are robust across investigators, settings, and subjects, indicating the high level of generalization that has been achieved with the treatment approach.

However, even when **treatment efficacy** has been established with a highly controlled group or single subject designs, there is still an element of risk in applying findings to an individual child. This important concern for demonstrating treatment efficacy with the individual is addressed in this book by introducing single subject design methodology in the later

Table 9–1 A Hierarchy of Treatment Efficacy Evidence: Guidelines for Selecting Treatment Procedures for Evidence-Based Practice

Level of Evidence	Research Method	Interpretation	Recommendation
Level 1 Expert Advocacy	None	No evidence to support advocated technique	Reject technique until positive evidence emerges
Level 2 Uncontrolled Unreplicated	A case study; not a controlled experiment	A claim of improvement but not effectiveness	Use technique only when no technique with higher level evidence is available
Level 3 Uncontrolled Directly Replicated	A case study that has been replicated by the same investigator	Reliability of the originally claimed improvement is shown	The same as level 2; the claimed improvement may be more reliable
Level 4 Uncontrolled Systematically Replicated	A case study that has been replicated by others in various settings	Greater generalizability of improvement is established	Same as level 3; the claimed improvement may be realized in different settings with the same technique
Level 5 Controlled Unreplicated	An experimental design of group or single subject design	Efficacy not just improvement can be claimed	Use with caution; watch for replications and contradictory evidence
Level 6 Controlled Directly Replicated	The same experimental design as in the original study implemented by original investigator	Reliability of originally claimed effectiveness is shown	Use technique with greater confidence; watch for replications and contradictory evidence
Level 7 Controlled Systematically Replicated	An experimental design implemented by different investigators in various settings	Generality of effectiveness is well established	Recommended for general professional practice

Source: Hedge and Maul, Language Disorders in Children, © 2006. Reproduced by permission of Pearson Education, Inc.

portion of this chapter. Beforehand, the literature is reviewed by describing treatment approaches in terms of the hierarchy of evidence presented in Table 9–1. This review has not considered every possible combination of factors: treatment activity by physical context by social context by etiological category by linguistic target because the number of possible combinations is staggering. Instead, the treatment procedure is emphasized, and the other factors are included as they present themselves. In addition, a case study that has been designed to demonstrate the intuitive value of EBP is provided.

EBT Literature Review

Clinician-Directed Approaches

The clinician-directed (CD) approaches are at the low end of the naturalness continuum. Hart and Risley (1980) reviewed the rich history of the CD approaches, which dates back to the 1950s. They noted that this early work in operant procedures revolutionized remedial training in language. More recently, this foundation has been elaborated on. The general reviews of the more recent literature of the CD approaches by Abbeduto and Boudreau (2004); Baldwin and Baldwin (1998); Camarata, Nelson, and Camarata, (1994); Fey (1986); Goldstein (2002); Hegde and Maul (2006); Malott, Malott, and Trojan (2000); Martin and Pear (1999); Nelson, Camarata, Welsh, Butkovsky, and Camarata (1996); Paul (2007); and Paul and Sutherland (2005) provide strong support for all of the clinical procedures described, including modeling, prompting, fading, reinforcing, instructing, shaping, and providing feedback. Paul (2007) pointed out that the CD approaches are characterized by an extensive empirical literature, which shows that they are effective over a wide variety of linguistic forms with a heterogeneous group of language-disordered children. Support for these treatment procedures is at the highest level in the hierarchy of evidence (Table 9–1).

There is a paucity of empirical support for teaching metalinguistic skills using the CD approaches. One exception is that Kaufman, Prelock, Weiler, Creaghead, and Donnelly (1994) increased metalinguistic awareness of explanatory adequacy in language-normal third graders. The researchers used a pretest–posttest control group design without random assignment of subjects to groups. In group designs, multiple subjects are included and a statistical analysis is generally completed. The pretest–posttest terminology indicates that group performance before and after treatment is compared. The control group is not treated to provide a contrast to the experimental group that is treated. However, not randomly assigning subjects to groups introduced ambiguity with regard to the equivalency of the groups. As such, the design was quasi-experimental. However, an even greater drawback was that the study did not include students with language impairments.

Another notable exception is that Ezell and Goldstein (1992) taught four mildly mentally retarded 9-year-olds to comprehend idiomatic expressions. The trainer taught the students to differentiate the literal versus the idiomatic contexts, and each student learned to comprehend the idioms in an average of 20 sessions. A multiple baseline across subjects across sets of idioms was used to demonstrate treatment effects. In single subject design studies, individual variability in behavior is examined across experimental conditions as a means of determining treatment efficacy. In the multiple baseline across subjects, experimental control is provided by treating one randomly selected subject before the other. When the treated subject improves but the untreated subject does not, then the evidence suggests that the treatment is effective. Similarly, in the multiple baseline across behaviors, experimental control is provided by treating one randomly selected behavior before the other. When the treated behavior improves but the untreated behavior does not improve, then the evidence suggests that the treatment is effective. Direct replication of the program was shown. Therefore, EBP for treatment of metalinguistic awareness is at level 2 and for teaching idioms is at level 6 in Table 9–1. Clearly, more research is needed in these areas.

Despite considerable support, the CD approaches have been criticized for being ill conceived and unnatural (Abbeduto & Boudreau, 2004; Hubbell, 1981; Gillum, Camarata, Nelson, & Camarata, 2003; Norris & Hoffman, 1993; Owens, 2010; Paul, 2007; Paul & Sutherland, 2005; Peterson, 2004). Norris and Hoffman (1993) argued that language is "whole," so it should not be subdivided into individual components, which is often seen in the CD approaches. Others (Abbeduto & Boudreau, 2004; Gillum et al., 2003; Owens, 2010; Peterson, 2004) have suggested that the artificial quality of the CD approaches is responsible for the minimal generalization of skills from the training environment to natural communicative contexts. Paul and Sutherland (2005) proposed that the CD approaches elicit a passive communicative style that interferes with language development.

CD approaches have been used successfully with such a wide range of language-disordered children that it is easier to name the types of children who have not benefited from them. Paul (2007) indicated that some language-disordered children may not be able to comply or adjust to the high degree of structure. These children included those who are obstinate or unassertive. However, obstinate and unassertive children may respond favorably to naturalistic approaches. Acknowledging the apparent shortcomings associated with the CD approaches, Fey (1986) suggested that it would be a mistake to assume that natural is better in an absolute sense. Rather, he indicated that natural is better only when the procedures employed are effective in helping children achieve their individual goals. Paradoxically, unnaturalness may actually be advantageous, he continued. History has already shown that many language-impaired children have difficulty extracting linguistic forms in natural contexts. They may actually need highly structured treatments to succeed. Furthermore, treatment time is used efficiently. No other approach elicits and reinforces as many responses per unit of time. Both Fey (1986) and Paul (2007) concluded that, despite the drawbacks, clinicians should have the CD approaches in their clinical armamentarium.

Client-Centered Approaches

Client-centered (CC) approaches are at the opposite end of the continuum from CD approaches. CC approaches are the most natural and least structured. In general, there is a lot of support for naturalistic approaches. For example, McLean and Cripe (1997) reviewed 39 intervention studies involving a heterogeneous group of children with language disorders. They reported strong evidence to support the efficacy of naturalistic approaches in both group and single subjects design investigations. Delprato (2001) surveyed the literature in language intervention in autism. He compared the CD approach to natural language training in six single subject design and two group design studies. The single subject design studies were either reversal or multiple baseline across subject strategies, and both group studies used random assignment across subjects, indicating the high-quality inclusionary criteria for the review. In a reversal design, a subject is trained during phase 1 and training is withheld in phase 2. When performance improves with training and falls off with the cessation of training, then treatment effectiveness has been shown. All eight of the studies demonstrated the superiority of the naturalistic approaches over the CD approaches.

However, CC approaches only represent a subset of the universe of naturalistic approaches. Reviewing the CC approaches is the focus of this portion of the chapter. Numerous investigators have established the efficacy of the **general stimulation** approach (Girolametto & Weitzman, 2006; Paul & Sutherland, 2005). Girolametto and Weitzman (2006) reviewed two controlled randomized trials related to "It Takes Two to Talk," the Hanen Program for Parents. The mothers acquired the requisite skills and were effective in promoting verbal interactions in their children. Paul and Sutherland (2005) completed a review of the intervention literature in autism. The single subject and small group design studies showed that the autistic children's imitation, joint attention, and social play all increased with the CC approaches. As with the aforementioned review, while the children's overall verbal interactions increased, they did not make progress with regard to specific linguistic forms. Therefore, the CC approaches represent EBP at the highest level in Table 9–1 for increasing overall verbal interaction, but they are not recommended for addressing specific target responses or individualized goals.

Hybrid Approaches

Recall that the hybrid approaches to intervention fall along the continuum of naturalness at intermediate positions. Theoretically, they take the best features from each end. That is, the hybrid approaches are presented within an enticing responsive environment that has been designed to elicit the child's responses in a naturalistic or conversational context. The clinician's verbal input reflects not only the child's developmental level but also the specific forms that have been targeted as individualized goals. Behavioral procedures such as modeling, prompting, and reinforcing may be used in concert with principles designed to promote generalization.

Several investigators have demonstrated the effectiveness of **focused stimulation** in promoting language development in language-delayed children (Fey, Cleave, Long, & Hughes, 1993; Girolametto & Weitzman, 2006; Lederer, 2001). In these studies, parents received training in focused stimulation and applied this technique with their children in dyads. The children were heterogeneous with respect to the etiologic factors contributing to their language delays and ranged in age from 24 to 70 months. Girolametto and Weitzman (2006) reviewed three randomized controlled trials, and Fey et al. (1993) completed a randomized controlled experimental study as well. Lederer (2001) completed a pretest–posttest group design. There is sufficient evidence based on these studies to conclude that focused stimulation represents EBP at the highest level in Table 9–1.

The effectiveness of **recast training** in the context of naturalistic conversation has been demonstrated over a wide range of linguistic targets (Camarata et al., 1994; Fey et al., 1993; Gillum et al., 2003; Nelson et al., 1996; Proctor-Williams, Fey, & Loeb, 2001; Robertson & Weismer, 1999; Schwartz, Chapman, Terrell, Prelock, & Rowan, 1985; Skarakis-Doyle & Murphy, 1995; Yoder, Spruytenburg, Edwards, & Davies, 1995). A heterogeneous group of language-impaired children received training in dyads in these studies. Fey et al. (1993) used a controlled randomized group trial. Robertson and Weismer (1999) employed a pretest–posttest control group design. Proctor-Williams et al. (2001) completed a pretest–posttest group study, and Yoder et al. (1995) used a multiple baseline across subjects. Camarata et al. (1994) used an alternating treatments group design to index treatment efficacy in children with specific language impairment. In an alternating treatments design, two or more interventions are compared with respect to efficacy by implementing both interventions during the training phase an equal number of times but in a counterbalanced or randomized fashion. When the target behavior associated with one of the interventions is superior to the other, the data suggest that the associated intervention has greater efficacy. Nelson et al. (1996) used a pretest–posttest quasi-experimental design, which showed that children with specific language impairment achieved gains associated with the treatment. Gillum et al. (2003) trained four preschool language-impaired children with poor pre-intervention imitation skills. The four children exhibited gains associated with recast treatment. **Vertical restructuring** is a specific variation of recasting, and its efficacy with language-impaired preschoolers has been supported in the literature. Schwartz et al. (1985) used a nonparametric pretest–posttest small-group design with a control group. Nonparametric designs employ statistics that do not make assumptions about the population. Skarakis-Doyle and Murphy (1995) employed an interactive additive single subject experimental design. This rather complex hybrid design included both reversal and multiple baseline across behaviors components. Overall, the sentence recast procedure represents EBP at the highest level in Table 9–1.

Milieu teaching refers to a general model of intervention that is effective in promoting language development over a wide range of linguistic targets with a wide variety of children exhibiting language disorders (Abbeduto & Boudreau, 2004; Hancock & Kaiser, 2002; Hart & Risley, 1980; Kaiser, Hancock, & Nietfeld, 2000; Warren et al., 2006;

Warren, McQuarter, & Rogers-Warren, 1984). One variation of the general model is called **enhanced milieu teaching (EMT)**, which has databased support. Kaiser et al. (2000) used a multiple baseline across dyads to demonstrate its treatment efficacy. Hancock and Kaiser (2002) used EMT and successfully taught three autistic preschoolers language forms. Abbeduto and Boudreau (2004) reviewed the literature and concluded that EMT is effective in promoting language development in both autism and mental retardation. Hart and Risley (1980) reviewed several of their studies and noted that **incidental teaching**, another variation of milieu teaching, was effective in facilitating language development in children with language disorders. They concluded that incidental teaching reinforces language use as a response class, which is important to language acquisition. Warren et al. (1984) used another variation of milieu teaching called **mand-model** to improve verbal responsiveness in three language-delayed, socially isolated preschoolers. A multiple baseline across subjects design indexed treatment effects. Warren et al. (2006) reviewed 11 studies supporting the efficacy of **prelinguistic milieu teaching (PMT)**. The review included large group randomized trials, longitudinal investigations, and multiple baseline studies. Longitudinal investigations examine the behavior of the same participants over time. Clearly, the general model of milieu teaching represents EBP at the highest level in Table 9–1.

Dialogic book reading provides an effective mechanism for promoting language development across a wide variety of language-impaired children (Crain-Thoreson & Dale, 1999; Dale, Crain-Thoreson, Notari-Syverson, & Cole, 1996; Hargrave & Senechal, 2000; Huebner, 2000; Yoder et al., 1995). Yoder et al. (1995) used a multiple baseline across subjects to demonstrate treatment efficacy. Dale et al. (1996) randomly assigned mother–child dyads to a dialogic reading group, where mothers were successful in improving the children's language. Crain-Thoreson and Dale (1999) reported language development in language-impaired children who participated in a dialogic reading program. They found that the more the adults increased their dialogic reading skills the more the children's scores improved in the pretest–posttest design study. Both Hargrave and Senechal (2000) and Huebner (2000) compared the effects of dialogic reading group with conventional reading in terms of language acquisition. Children in the conventional reading group showed improved language in both studies, but those in the dialogic reading groups improved more. Overall, dialogic reading represents EBP at the highest level in Table 9–1.

Script training may serve as a model to promote a variety of social interactions, such as conversational, narrative, and classroom discourse (Hegde & Maul, 2006). Numerous investigators have found that **script training** increases social interaction in the language-impaired population (Goldstein & Cisar, 1992; Gronna, Serna, Kennedy, & Prater, 1999; Krantz & McClannahan, 1998; Robertson & Weismer, 1997; Sarakoff, Taylor, & Poulson, 2001). Robertson and Weismer (1997) integrated two studies: a randomized pretest–posttest control group design plus a multiple baseline across subjects that partially replicated the first study. Both Krantz and McClannahan (1998) and Sarokoff et al. (2001) used a multiple baseline across subjects to evidence the effectiveness of a script-fading procedure. Goldstein and Cisar (1992) demonstrated the efficacy of script training by means of a multiple baseline across scripts, replicated across triads. Gronna et al. (1999) used a script training procedure with a visually impaired preschooler. A multiple baseline across skills, replicated across scripts, was used to illuminate treatment efficacy. Overall, it is apparent that script training meets EBP criteria at the highest level in Table 9–1.

Case Study

The following hypothetical case study was devised to demonstrate the value of EBP on a more intuitive level. It places a speech-language pathologist in a critical professional role in which relying on EBP is helpful in making a professional judgment in the context of a complex and emotional human drama. Recall that EBP seeks to integrate research evidence and clinical expertise with patient values.

Marcus, a nonspeaking 4-year-old profoundly impaired male diagnosed with an autism spectrum disorder (ASD) and childhood apraxia of speech (CAS), was scheduled to be seen at the Echo Speech and Hearing Clinic. The purpose of the appointment was to initiate treatment planning to enhance Marcus's communicative proficiency.

Marcus's mother, Crystal, explained on the preinterview questionnaire that she believed that Marcus was autistic because of her deficient parenting skills and that she felt personally responsible for her son's severe impairment. Moreover, she had learned on Google that facilitated communication (FC) would be helpful. Crystal had been greatly relieved to find out that FC was designed to help children with autism, mental retardation, and apraxia. She had learned that in FC the facilitator provides manual support for the impaired child's arm at a keyboard, which facilitates the child's undisclosed literacy and capacity for symbolic communication. Moreover, she could expect startling results with FC. Therefore, she was interested in having the speech-language pathologist at Echo implement a program of FC.

Marge, a speech-language pathologist, was assigned as the clinician at Echo. After reading the questionnaire, Marge completed a literature review of FC because she had not previously used the intervention procedure although she had heard of it. She found out that there was apparently some legitimate interest in FC back in the 1980s, but by the end of the 1990s, FC had been generally discredited. Today, although a few holdouts continue to advocate for FC, the empirical studies tend to suggest that the facilitator was unintentionally cueing the person. Interestingly, the more empirical the study, the more likely it was to discount the value of FC. Proponents of FC provided support using either anecdotal evidence or uncontrolled case studies. Marge accepted the databased evidence over the anecdotes and expert opinion and made a professional judgment against implementing FC.

Marge decided that she would acknowledge and try to channel the energy that Crystal had for helping her son. She would attempt to enlist Crystal as a teammate to explore the best possible ways of helping Marcus. She wanted to avoid sounding like a know-it-all, which may interfere with developing a helping relationship. Marge designed a three-pronged strategy. First, she would share information with Crystal that shows that today autism is regarded as having an organic or biologic basis and that most professionals no longer believe that autism is caused by poor parenting. Second, she would provide additional and more balanced information on FC so that it would become apparent to Crystal that her information was biased. Third, she would review the current approaches to intervention in autism with Crystal, emphasizing the important role of the parent in the intervention program. Once Crystal agreed, they would implement a program of treatment together.

Single Subject Design

Single subject design (SSD) refers to a methodology that focuses on individual variability under experimental conditions as a means of attributing the change in the **dependent variable (DV)**, the targets to the **independent variable (IV)**, the treatments. Clearly, this is of great concern to the clinician who values EBP. SSD has been described more fully elsewhere (e.g., Hegde, 1994). As shown in **Figure 9–1**, by convention, the quality of performance, generically referred to here as number of target

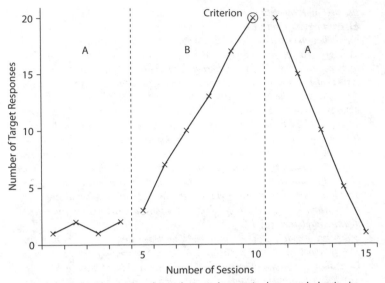

Figure 9–1 The A-B-A single subject design where a single target behavior is taught to a single individual using a single treatment program.

responses, is shown on the y-axis, and the number of sessions across time is indicated on the x-axis. Vertical lines divide the sessions into phases, where A represents the baseline phase and B represents the treatment phase, which is followed here by another A phase. Data points are connected within phases to emphasize the cohesive nature of a phase. As shown, the DV is measured repeatedly under different experimental conditions and depicted in xy space for visual inspection and interpretation.

In the A-B-A design, a particular SSD, the experimenter first measures the DV in the baseline phase a sufficient number of times so that its inherent variability can be observed. If there is a positive trend, then the baseline phase needs to be continued until it stabilizes. Then, the treatment phase is initiated, and the DV continues to be measured and graphed. The B phase continues until criterion is met. After criterion has been met, the experimenter introduces another A phase, where the DV is measured in the same manner as the initial A phase. The only factor that is allowed to change between adjacent phases is the treatment so its influence may be examined.

To illustrate how the findings are interpreted by visual inspection, assume the experimenter achieved the results shown in Figure 9–1. Performance has been idealized for clarity. In the initial baseline phase, performance was stable and at a low level. When treatment was implemented, performance improved to a high level and criterion was met in session 10. Then, the second baseline phase was initiated and a reversal of the positive trend was apparent as performance deteriorated. Noting that performance only improved with the onset of treatment and fell off when treatment ceased, the most parsimonious interpretation was that the treatment was responsible for the changes in the target behavior. However, had performance not deteriorated with the cessation of treatment, then experimental control would have been lost and the improvement associated with the treatment could not have been attributed to the treatment.

The A-B-A design should only be employed with a DV expected to deteriorate with the cessation of treatment. Otherwise, treatment efficacy cannot be demonstrated with this design. As such, the general stimulation procedure for increasing verbal communication may be a good candidate to use with the A-B-A design. The specific question to be addressed in this hypothetical example is whether an increase in verbal communication for this child can be attributed to the general stimulation condition in contrast to a free-play condition. In the initial A phase, the child's spontaneous utterances are counted during 15-minute periods in the free-play condition. In free play, the clinician simply sets out some play materials and interacts with the child in an unstructured fashion. During B phase, the child's spontaneous utterances are counted for 15-minute periods in the general stimulation condition. During general stimulation, the clinician enables the child to select the materials and provides a responsive environment that includes parallel play, self-talk, and treating the child's utterances as if they were communicative even if they were not. Then, in the second A phase, the clinician counts the child's spontaneous utterances in the same manner as in the initial A phase. The hypothetical data in Figure 9–1 provide strong support that indicates that the general stimulation condition increased verbal communication over the free-play condition.

The multiple baseline across behavior SSD is superior to the A-B-A design for demonstrating treatment efficacy with a DV, which is not expected to fall off with the cessation of treatment. This design is depicted in **Figure 9–2**. Here, two different target behaviors are sequentially

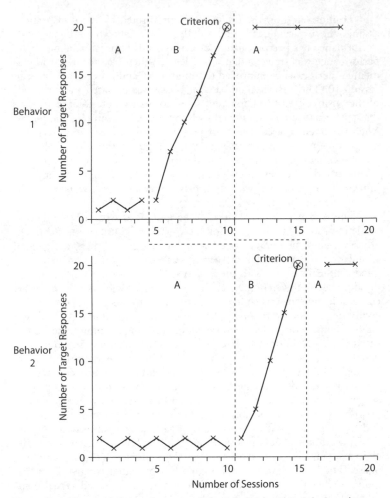

Figure 9–2 The multiple baseline across behaviors single subject design where two target behaviors are sequentially taught to a single individual using a single treatment program.

taught to a single subject using a single treatment procedure. One of the targets is randomly selected to be taught first.

As shown in Figure 9–2, after baselining behavior 1 to demonstrate pretreatment stability and a low level of performance, treatment on behavior 1 is initiated, while behavior 2 continues to be baselined. During the treatment phase, behavior 1 exhibits a positive trend and reaches criterion during session 10, at which time the treatment phase is terminated and the second baseline phase is initiated. For behavior 2, pretreatment performance is at a low level and stable. Treatment is initiated after criterion has been met on behavior 1. A positive trend is exhibited in behavior 2 and criterion is met in session 15. During the second baseline phase, performance remained at a high level for both behaviors.

The idealized data presented in Figure 9–2 would be interpreted as follows: Pretreatment performance was stable and at a low level for both behaviors. Improvements only occurred in behavior 1 and subsequently in behavior 2 when treatment was applied to those particular behaviors, respectively. Therefore, the most parsimonious interpretation was that the treatment was responsible for the improvement. However, if during the treatment of behavior 1, behavior 2 had improved, then experimental control would have been lost and the improvement associated with the treatment could not have been attributed to the treatment. The important point is that each behavior only improved when treatment was applied specifically to it.

The multiple baseline across behaviors SSD is effective in demonstrating treatment efficacy over a wide range of treatments. As a hypothetical example, a single treatment package consisting of focused stimulation plus recasting will be used to train two target behaviors: (1) verbally producing the auxiliary verb *is* as in *He is running* and (2) verbally producing the locative prepositions (*in, on, under, over*), as in *The ball is on the table*. Baselining occurs in a free-play condition in a clinician–child dyad. Free play lasts 15 minutes. During this period, the clinician makes available a variety of play objects and interacts with the child in an unstructured fashion. The clinician counts the number of instances that the child spontaneously utters each of the two target forms but refrains from modeling and recasting. In the treatment condition, the clinician uses selected materials to elicit the target behavior. The clinician models the target form repeatedly in a meaningful communicative context and waits expectantly for a response. When a response is elicited, the clinician imitates the response when it is correct and recasts it when it is deficient. The target behavior is baselined in the exact same manner in all probe conditions, that is, in the pretreatment baseline, after each treatment session and after treatment has been terminated. Therefore, the data of interest are not the training data but those data reflecting generalization of the target behaviors to the free-play condition. As indicated in Figure 9–2, the hypothetical data strongly support the hypothesis that the treatment package was effective in training the target responses.

Chapter Summary

Evidence-based practice is introduced as a guiding principle for the management of children diagnosed with language disorders. Each of the major approaches to treating language disorders is described with regard to a hierarchy of treatment efficacy evidence. Principles of single subject design methodology are presented to provide clinicians with a vehicle for demonstrating treatment efficacy of a treatment plan with an individual child.

Terms from the Chapter

Controlled investigations *(152)*
Dependent variable *(161)*
Dialogic book reading *(159)*
Direct replication *(152)*
Enhanced milieu teaching *(159)*
Evidence-based practice *(151)*
Expert opinion *(152)*
Focused stimulation *(157)*
General stimulation *(157)*
Incidental teaching *(159)*
Independent variable *(161)*

Mand-model *(159)*
Milieu teaching *(158)*
Peer reviewed *(152)*
Prelinguistic milieu teaching *(159)*
Recast training *(158)*
Script training *(160)*
Single subject design *(161)*
Systematic replication *(152)*
Treatment efficacy *(152)*
Uncontrolled investigations *(152)*
Vertical restructuring *(158)*

References

Abbeduto, L., & Boudreau, D. (2004). Theoretical influences in research on language development and intervention in individuals with mental retardation. *Mental Retardation and Developmental Disabilities Research Reviews, 10*, 184–192.

American Speech-Language-Hearing Association. (2004). *Evidence-based practice in communication disorders: An introduction* [Technical report]. Retrieved from www.asha.org/policy

Baldwin, J. D., & Baldwin, J. I. (1998). *Behavioral principles in everyday life* (3rd ed.). Upper Saddle River, NJ: Prentice Hall.

Camarata, S. M., Nelson, K. E., & Camarata, M. (1994). Comparison of conversational recasting and imitative procedures for training grammatical structures in children with specific language impairment. *Journal of Speech and Hearing Research, 37*, 1414–1423.

Crain-Thoreson, C., & Dale, P. S. (1999). Enhancing linguistic performance: Parents and teachers as book reading partners for children with language delays. *Topics in Early Childhood Special Education, 19*, 28–40.

Dale, P., Crain-Thoreson, C., Notari-Syverson, A., & Cole, K. (1996). Parent-child story-book reading as an intervention technique for young children with language delays. *Topics in Early Childhood Special Education, 16*, 213–235.

Delprato, D. (2001). Comparison of discrete-trial and normalized behavioral language intervention for young children with autism. *Journal of Autism and Developmental Disorders, 31*, 315–325.

Ezell, H. K., & Goldstein, H. (1992). Teaching idiom comprehension to children with mental retardation. *Journal of Applied Behavior Analysis, 25*, 181–191.

Fey, M. E. (1986). *Language intervention in young children.* San Diego, CA: College Hill Press.

Fey, M. E., Cleave, P. L., Long, S. H., & Hughes, D. L. (1993). Two approaches to facilitation of grammar in language impaired children: An experimental evaluation. *Journal of Speech and Hearing Research, 36*, 141–157.

Gillum, H., Camarata, S., Nelson, K. E., & Camarata, M. N. (2003). A comparison of naturalistic and analog treatment effects in children with expressive language disorder and poor pre-intervention skills. *Journal of Positive Behavior Interventions, 5*, 171–178.

Girolametto, L., & Weitzman, E. (2006). It takes two to talk: The Hanen Program for Parents. In R. McCauley & M. Fey (Eds.), *Treatment of language disorders in children* (pp. 77–101). Baltimore, MD: Paul H. Brookes.

Goldstein, H. (2002). Communication intervention for children with autism: A review of treatment efficacy. *Journal of Autism and Developmental Disorders, 32*, 373–396.

Goldstein, H., & Cisar, C. L. (1992). Promoting interaction during sociodramatic play: Teaching scripts to typical preschoolers and classmates with disabilities. *Journal of Applied Behavior Analysis, 25*, 265–280.

Gronna, S. S., Serna, L. A., Kennedy, C. H., & Prater, M. A. (1999). Promoting generalized social interactions using puppets and script training in an integrated preschool: A single case study using multiple baseline design. *Behavior Modification, 23*, 419–440.

Hancock, T. B., & Kaiser, A. P. (2002). The effects of trainer-implemented enhanced milieu teaching on social communication of children with autism. *Topics in Early Childhood Special Education, 22*, 39–55.

Hargrave, H., & Senechal, M. (2000). Book reading intervention with preschool children who have limited vocabularies: The benefits of regular reading and dialogic reading. *Early Childhood Research Quarterly, 15*, 75–90.

Hart, B. & Risley, T. (1980). In vivo language intervention: Unanticipated general effects. *Journal of Applied Behavior Analysis, 13*, 407–432.

Hegde, M. N. (1994). *Clinical research in communication disorders: Principles and strategies* (2nd ed.). Austin, TX: PRO-ED.

Hegde, M. N., & Maul, C. A. (2006). *Language disorders in children: An evidence-based approach to assessment and treatment.* Boston, MA: Pearson Education.

Hubbell, R. (1981). *Children's language disorders: An integrated approach.* Englewood Cliffs, NJ: Prentice Hall.

Huebner, C. (2000). Promoting toddler's language development through community based intervention. *Journal of Applied Developmental Psychology, 21*, 513–535.

Kaiser, A. P., Hancock, T. B., & Nietfeld, J. P. (2000). The effects of parent-implemented enhanced milieu teaching on social communication of children who have autism. *Early Education and Development, 11*, 423–446.

Kaufman, S. S., Prelock, P. A., Weiler, E. M., Creaghead, N. A., & Donnelly, C. A. (1994). Metapragmatic awareness of explanatory adequacy: Developing skills for academic success from a collaborative communication skills unit. *Language, Speech and Hearing Services in Schools, 25*, 174–180.

Krantz, P. J., & McClannahan, L. E. (1998). Social interaction skills for children with autism: A script-fading procedure for beginning readers. *Journal of Applied Behavior Analysis, 31*, 191–202.

Lederer, S. H. (2001). Efficacy of parent-child language group intervention for late-talking toddlers. *Infant-Toddler Intervention, 11*, 223–235.

Malott, R. W., Malott, M. E., & Trojan, E. A. (2000). *Elementary principles of behavior* (4th ed.). Upper Saddle River, NJ: Prentice Hall.

Martin, G., & Pear, J. (1999). *Behavior modification: What it is and how to do it* (6th ed.). Upper Saddle River, NJ: Prentice Hall.

McLean, L., & Cripe, J. (1997). The effectiveness of early intervention for children with communication disorders. In M. Guralnick (Ed.), *The effectiveness of early intervention* (pp. 349–428). Baltimore, MD: Paul H. Brookes.

Nelson, K. E., Camarata, S. M., Welsh, J., Butkovsky, L., & Camarata, M. (1996). Effects of imitation and conversational recasting treatment on the acquisition of grammar in children with specific language impairment and younger language-normal children. *Journal of Speech and Hearing Research, 39*, 850–859.

Norris, J., & Hoffman, P. (1993). *Whole language intervention for school age children.* San Diego, CA: Singular Publishing.

Owens, R. E. (2010). *Language disorders: A functional approach to assessment and intervention* (5th ed.). Boston, MA: Pearson.

Paul, R. (2007). *Language disorders from infancy through adolescence: Assessment and intervention* (3rd ed.). St. Louis, MO: Mosby.

Paul, R., & Sutherland, D. (2005). Enhancing early language in children with autism spectrum disorders. In F. Volkmar, R. Paul, A. King, & D. Cohen (Eds.), *Handbook of autism and pervasive developmental disorders* (Vol. 2, pp. 946–976). New York, NY: Wiley.

Peterson, P. (2004). Naturalistic language teaching procedures for children at risk for language delays. *Behavioral Analyst Today*, *5*, 404–424.

Proctor-Williams, K., Fey, M., & Loeb, D. (2001). Parental recasts and production of copulas and articles by children with specific language impairment and typical development. *American Journal of Speech Language Pathology*, *10*, 155–168.

Robertson, S. B., & Weismer, S. E. (1997). The influence of peer models on play scripts of children with specific language impairment. *Journal of Speech, Language and Hearing Research*, *40*, 49–61.

Robertson, S. E., & Weismer, S. E. (1999). Effects of treatment on linguistic and social skills in toddlers with delayed language development. *Journal of Speech, Language and Hearing Research*, *42*, 1234–1248.

Sackett, D. L., Straus, S. E., Richardson, W. S., Rosenberg, W., & Haynes, R. B. (2000). *Evidence based medicine: How to practice and teach EBM* (2nd ed.). New York, NY: Churchill Livingstone.

Sarakoff, R. A., Taylor, B. A., & Poulson, C. L. (2001). Teaching children with autism to engage in conversational exchanges: Script fading with embedded textual stimuli. *Journal of Applied Behavior Analysis*, *34*, 81–84.

Schwartz, R., Chapman, K., Terrell, B., Prelock, P., & Rowan, L. (1985). Facilitating word combinations in language-impaired children through discourse structure. *Journal of Speech and Hearing Disorders*, *50*, 31–39.

Skarakis-Doyle, E., & Murphy, L. (1995). Discourse-based language intervention: An efficacy study. *Journal of Children's Communication Development*, *17*, 11–22.

Warren, S., Bredin-Oja, S., Fairchild, M., Finestack, L., Fey, M., & Brady, N. (2006). Responsivity education: Prelinguistic milieu teaching. In R. McCauley & M. Fey (Eds.), *Treatment of language disorders in children* (pp. 47–75). Baltimore, MD: Paul H. Brookes.

Warren, S., McQuarter, R., & Rogers-Warren, A. (1984). The effects of mands and models on the speech of unresponsive language delayed preschool children. *Journal of Speech and Hearing Disorders*, *49*, 43–52.

Yoder, P. J., Spruytenburg, H., Edwards, A., & Davies, B. (1995). Effect of verbal routine contexts and expansions on gains in mean length of utterance in children with developmental delays. *Language, Speech and Hearing Services in Schools*, *26*, 21–32.

EVIDENCE-BASED PRACTICE

CHAPTER 10

Exemplars of Intervention Procedures

*Ronald B. Hoodin, Bill Cupples, Linda J. Polter,
Denise Kowalski, Brenda Doster, Ana Claudia Harten,
and Lizbeth Curme Stevens*

Chapter Objectives

After reading this chapter, you should be able to

- Define the concept of an exemplar.
- Discuss how an exemplar may be modified.
- Explain how relevant exemplars are identified using Tables 10–1 and 10–2.

This final chapter is a culmination of all of the preceding chapters of the handbook. It provides exemplars, or examples, of treatment procedures to serve as models for intervention. The exemplars reflect a wide range of treatments with respect to age of the child, modality to be trained, linguistic parameter to be addressed, level of intervention, and type of treatment, as well as special features, such as sensitivity to multicultural issues. Each exemplar has been written following a generic format to add clarity and reduce complexity. Each has been numbered to facilitate referencing. The target behavior to be taught is defined conceptually to orient the reader and defined operationally to add specificity.

The treatment is described in a systematic fashion. Each exemplar is described with respect to the training environment, the materials to be used, and the roles of the clinician and child. Every exemplar makes assumptions about the child's level. Therefore, each is also described with respect to the recommended preparation of the child for the activities. Finally, the author of the exemplar provides additional clinical insights for using the exemplar that have not otherwise been addressed. Exemplar 0 has been included to provide further information of the generic format used with all of the exemplars.

Modifying the Exemplars

The exemplars in this chapter are prototypical. That is, each **exemplar** simultaneously serves as an example of a particular treatment that may be implemented in its present form, and each exemplar represents a type of treatment that may be modified in some way before being implemented. For example, one exemplar may describe treatment with an individual child. It also may be modified based on clinical judgment so that it is used in a small group or even in a classroom assignment. Another exemplar may describe training the regular plural morpheme in receptive language and the clinician may choose to modify the exemplar so that it can be implemented to train the same morpheme expressively. Modifications may also be made with respect to target behaviors. That is, an exemplar may describe how to teach a child to use requesting. The clinician may draw on his or her judgment to modify the exemplar to teach the child another conversational skill, such as commenting. An exemplar may be modified to accommodate a child's impairment. For example, a clinician who is working with a hearing-impaired child may choose to modify the environment by ensuing a low ambient noise level, that faces are illuminated, and that individuals speak clearly while facing the child. As such, while 30 different exemplars have been presented in this chapter, the clinician can make these modifications to significantly multiply their applications. Practice facilitates the skill of modification and is encouraged accordingly.

The Tables

Table 10–1 has been designed to help the reader identify relevant exemplars in a straightforward and efficient manner. As shown in Table 10–1, the exemplars have been classified according to variables that are salient to the clinician. The table lists the variables of interest and their associated codes in the first two columns. The reader enters the table based on these variables. The third column identifies the associated exemplars by number. The exemplar number references a particular exemplar. The exemplars are sequenced in general based on when the target behavior would show up in the child's chronological development. As such, exemplars for infants appear at the beginning, whereas those involving

Table 10–1 Identifying Relevant Exemplars Based on Salient Variables

Variable	Subcategory/ Abbreviation	Exemplar
Age of Child	Infant (In)	1,2
	Toddler (Td)	1,3,4,5,6,7
	Preschool (PSc)	4,6,7,8,9,10,11,12,13,14,15,16
	School (Sc)	4,5,6,7,11,12,13,14,15,16,17,18,19, 20,21,22,23,24,25,26,27,28,29,30
Modality to Be Trained	Receptive (Rc)	4,6,11,12,15,21,22,25,26,27,28,29,30
	Expressive (Ex)	1,2,3,4,5,7,8,9,10,13,14,15,16, 17,18,19,20,22,23,24,27,29,30
Parameter to Be Trained	Semantic (Se)	21,22,4,25,26,15,27,28,29,5,6
	Syntactic (Sn)	5,8,9,10,12,16,17,18,19,20,27,28
	Morphologic (Mr)	8,9,10,11,12,16,17,18,19,20,27,28
	Pragmatic (Pr)	1,2,3,5,6,7,13,14,23,24,27,29,30
Level of Intervention	Acquisition (Ac)	1,2,4,5,6,7,8,9,10,11,12,13,15,16, 17,18,21,22,23,25,26,27,28,29,30
	Generalization (Gn)	19,20,14,24
Type of Intervention	Clinician directed (CD)	8,9,10,11,12,15,16,17,18, 19,20,21,22,26,27,28
	Client centered (CC)	3,2
	Hybrid (Hb)	4,5,6,7,13,14,23,24,25,29,30
Special Features	Advanced language (AL)	17,18,19,21,22,12,23, 24,25,26,27,28,29,30
	Multicultural (Mc)	15,27
	Aug/Alt communication (AAC)	6,7

advanced language targets are positioned at the end. Otherwise, the number has no particular meaning. Once the exemplar of interest has been identified, the reader goes to the actual exemplar. The exemplars are presented in numerical order. Of course, the reader is not obliged to use the table. The reader, who is so inclined, may simply browse through the exemplars. However, the exemplars have not really been designed to be read sequentially, page after page, as in a typical chapter. Doing so may be tedious. Use of the table is strategic in that regard.

Table 10–2 Target Behaviors Associated with Each Exemplar

Exemplar	Target Behavior	Exemplar	Target Behavior
1	Preintentional social interaction	16	Noun phrases
2	Joint attention	17	Gerunds
3	Overall verbal interaction	18	Infinitives
4	Animal vocabulary	19	Gerunds—generalized
5	Requesting	20	Infinitives—generalized
6	Symbolization in AAC	21	Awareness of metaphors
7	Communication in AAC	22	Explaining metaphors
8	Present progressive	23	Personal narratives
9	Regular past tense	24	Narratives—generalized
10	Future tense	25	Awareness of idioms—I
11	Regular plural	26	Awareness of idioms—II
12	Count and mass nouns	27	Curriculum-based narratives
13	Appropriate eye contact	28	Auxiliary verbs
14	Eye contact—generalized	29	Expository text
15	Prepositions	30	Story grammar

AAC = augmentative/alternative communication.

Table 10–2 lists the various target behaviors associated with the exemplars. It provides an overview. As such, if the reader were interested a particular target behavior, for example, gerunds, he or she may simply scan the list in this table and readily see that exemplars 17 and 19 should be reviewed.

Exemplar 0

Explanation of Generic Format for Exemplars

Conceptually Define the Target Behavior: Tells the target behavior in conceptual terms.

Operationally Define the Treatment: Indicates what the child will do (correct response) using empirical, measurable, objective terms in what conditions specifying the environment, materials, and stimulus conditions, including contingent consequences, and tells the criteria for mastery.

> **Environment**: Describes the environment or environmental modifications for treatment; for example, an elementary school classroom with rows of seats and desks or sitting with a child on a carpeted floor.

> **Materials**: Describes any materials used; for example, photographs of family members or everyday objects including shoes, balls, and so on.

> **Stimulus Conditions**: Describes what the clinician does, including presentation of the materials, the use of models, prompts, cues, reinforcement, and feedback.

Preparation: Explains what the clinician may have to do to prepare the child to participate in the task; for example, being sure that the child understands the vocabulary words that are used in the activity.

Other Clinical Considerations: Provides additional insights associated with the exemplar that have not already been covered but which may be relevant; for example, telling the next logical step after mastery has been met on the current target behavior.

Codes: At the end of each exemplar is a list of codes that indicates salient features that characterize the particular exemplar. The codes for approximate age of the child are as follows: infant (In), toddler (Td), preschool aged, (PSc) and school aged (Sc); for modality trained: receptive (Rc) and expressive (Ex); for linguistic parameter involved: semantic (Se), syntactic (Sn), morphologic (Mr), and pragmatic (Pr); for level: acquisition (Ac) and generalization (Gn); for type of treatment: clinician directed (CD), client centered (CC), and hybrid (Hb); as well as for special features, including advanced language (AL) and multicultural sensitivity (Mc), and augmentative/alternative communication (AAC).

Exemplar 1

Ronald B. Hoodin

Conceptually Define the Target Behavior: Increased early vocalization will be trained as preintentional social interaction.

Operationally Define the Treatment: The infant/toddler will spontaneously vocalize or vocalize in response to a model provided in the context of an enticing supportive context 80 percent of the time.

> **Environment**: The interaction will occur when the child is in his or her crib, playpen, or other such place from time to time throughout the day.
>
> **Material**: None.
>
> **Stimulus Conditions**: The clinician will come up close to the child, get in the child's line of sight, and move a body part as necessary to get the child's attention. When the child spontaneously vocalizes, the clinician will treat him as if he were communicative even if he were not. The clinician will imitate the vocalization and provide reinforcement (e.g., talking in an animated fashion; picking up, hugging, or caressing the infant; providing juice). If the child does not spontaneously vocalize, the clinician models cooing (vocalizing coupled with the production of consonants produced in the posterior oral cavity, such as *k* and *g*) or babbling (vocalizing using a variety of different consonants, such as *ba ba ba*) and waits expectantly for a vocal response. When one occurs, the clinician imitates it and provides reinforcement. If none occurs, another model is provided.

Preparation: The clinician should refrain from providing treatment when the infant is overly stimulated or distressed. Signs of overstimulation in infants include irritability, irregular breathing, jerky movements, dull gaze, and pale or ashen skin color. Rather, the clinician should provide treatment when the child is relaxed, positioned on his or her back, satiated, happy, playful, and responsive. The clinician may have to check at various times throughout the day to determine the best times to provide treatment.

Other Clinical Considerations: The intervention described here reflects many of the ideas from Hegde and Maul (2006). While this early social–communicative interaction is regarded as preintentional, it is not limited to vocalizations and may include eye contact, body movements, or gestures. These early interactions may provide a foundation for later-emerging clear, frequent, prelinguistic, intentional communication, which is also multimodal in nature and provides a basis for the subsequent use of words and multiword utterances when the child begins to acquire spoken language.

Codes: In, Td, Ex, Pr, Ac, Hb.

Reference

Hegde, M. N., & Maul, C. A. (2006). *Language disorders in children: An evidence-based approach to assessment and treatment*. Boston, MA: Pearson Education.

Exemplar 2

Bill Cupples

Conceptually Define the Target Behavior: Pointing to establish joint attention to request will be trained.

Operationally Define the Treatment: The child will point to a desired object out of reach to request it and establish eye contact with the clinician five times.

> **Environment**: Intervention will occur in a well-lit, quiet room with the clinician and the child sitting on the floor.
>
> **Materials**: A variety of toys will be arranged in a naturalistic play setting around the room, in sight but out of reach. Some will be hanging in plastic zipper bags, some on shelves in sight. Caregivers have been consulted to determine which toys or objects would be most desirable for the child.
>
> **Stimulus Conditions**: The clinician will direct the child's attention to the toys by pointing and commenting. The clinician will follow the child's lead by following the child's gaze and commenting on the toys the child is gazing at. When the child reaches, the clinician will take the child's hand and shape it to a point. When a point occurs, the child will receive the toy to play with. Each toy will have a component part in another location. As the child plays with the toy, the clinician directs the child's attention to the component part, encouraging pointing to request the additional part. When the child points, the clinician will retrieve the toy for the child to play with.

Preparation: Before seeing the child, the clinician will have consulted with caregivers to determine which toys will be desirable. Toys will be arranged around the room in sight but inaccessible to the child. Some toys will be in plastic zipper bags, some on shelves, and some in clear plastic containers.

Code: In, Ex, Pr, Ac, CC.

Exemplar 3

Ronald B. Hoodin

Conceptually Define the Target Behavior: Increasing overall verbal interaction will be trained.

Operationally Define the Treatment: The child will verbally produce more spontaneous utterances when he or she is provided with an enticing environment.

> **Environment**: Intervention will occur in a quiet room with the child and clinician sitting side-by-side on a carpeted floor.

> **Materials**: Choices or alternative play materials (e.g., blocks, cars) are presented, from which the child makes a selection.

> **Stimulus Conditions**: The clinician engages in parallel play with the child so they are both playing with the materials that the child selected. Then, the clinician begins the general stimulation procedure. That is, the clinician starts talking about what he/she is doing so that the child can see a close match between the clinician's words and actions (e.g., *I am making the car go. The car is going. See the car go.*). The child will likely attend to the clinician because after all, the child selected the materials, suggesting that the activity is of interest. Furthermore, the clinician speaks in an animated fashion to attract the child's notice. In this fashion, the clinician provides a model for imitation although no demands are made on the child. After providing the model, the clinician waits expectantly for the child to respond. When the child responds, the clinician treats the child's behavior as meaningful and communicative, even if it were not. When the child responds verbally, the clinician imitates the child. Even though the child is not required to imitate, it is likely that the child will imitate the imitation. When the child does imitate, this may encourage a turn-taking-type dialogue. Children often imitate adult models, so taken together these techniques maximize the chance that the child will make a spontaneous utterance.

Preparation: No specific preparation is required. This approach has been designed for children who are young, immature, passive, or unable to comply with the structure associated with other approaches to intervention.

Other Clinical Considerations: This approach is not capable of addressing specific language goals. Since no demands are made on the child, the child does not use his or her energies to resist. Instead, the child may respond in a more natural fashion. Therefore, this is a good starting point. When the child reaches the level of regularly contributing to conversations, the clinician should change approaches so that individual goals are addressed.

Codes: Td, Ex, Pr, CC.

Exemplar 4

Ronald B. Hoodin

Conceptually Define the Target Behavior: In general, the vocabulary associated with animals will be trained.

Operationally Define the Treatment: The child will point to 10 pictures of animals, label 10 pictures of animals, and make 10 descriptive statements about what animals are doing in pictures.

> **Environment**: Intervention will occur in a quiet, well-lit room with the child and clinician sitting side-by-side on a couch.

> **Materials**: A child's book, based on the child's developmental level, good pictures of animals doing various activities (walking, running, flying, swimming, etc.), as well as a simple, straightforward narrative should be selected from an array of children's books.

> **Stimulus Conditions**: The clinician reads the storybook to the child each day so that the information becomes a shared experience. As the clinician reads the story, the child is encouraged to participate in this dialogic reading task. Initially, the clinician prompts the child to point to pictures describing the story. Later, the child answers questions about the story and the pictures. The clinician recasts the responses and engages the child in a dialogue about the story. Gradually, the child assumes the greater burden of telling the story while the clinician's role is relegated to providing prompts and support.

Preparation: In general, the clinician should try to interest the child in books to motivate the child to participate. Emphasis may be placed on showing enticing pictures and the idea that fascinating stories are held within the pages of books.

Other Clinical Considerations: The clinician may start dialogic book reading with one book but be on the lookout for other books that would be appropriate based on the child's developmental level, interest, and experiences. Dialogic book reading represents an excellent opportunity for parent involvement after the clinician trains them.

Codes: Td, PSc, Sc, Rc, Ex, Se Ac, Hb.

Exemplar 5

Bill Cupples

Conceptually Define the Target Behavior: The use of two-word phrases to request will be taught.

Operationally Define the Treatment: The child will say two-word phrases to request objects and actions using (agent + action) and (action + object), the semantic relationships, with 90 percent accuracy.

> **Environment**: Intervention will take place in a naturalistic play setting.
>
> **Materials**: Various age-appropriate toys are placed on the floor and on shelves out of reach.
>
> **Stimulus Condition**: The clinician will focus the child's attention on the out-of-reach toys or snacks. As the child gestures toward a toy, the clinician will model the appropriate phrase to request (e.g., *give truck*, *mommy give*). When the child produces the desired phrase, the clinician reinforces the request by handing the toy to the child.

Preparation: The clinician arranges various toys around the room out of reach but within the child's line of sight. Snacks are in plastic jars with lids on tight.

Other Clinical Considerations: A caregiver may be trained in this task by initially observing through a one-way mirror and, after a point, participating in the activity.

Codes: Td, PSc, Ex, Se, Sn, Pr, Ac, Hb.

Exemplar 6

Lizbeth Curme Stevens

Conceptually Define the Target Behavior: The child will associate a symbol with its referent.

Operationally Define the Treatment: The child will select a symbol to indicate a referent from an array of two symbols by pointing or touching with 90 percent accuracy.

> **Environment**: Intervention should take place during natural occurring routines. For example, symbols to be taught may be placed within the child's reach on a table in proximity to the referent during meals or on the floor during play.

> **Materials**: Target symbols selected for training (e.g., photographs, line drawings, actual objects, parts of an objects) should be for referents familiar to the child that are highly desirable or preferred and should be easy for the child to learn.

> **Stimulus conditions**: The clinician will follow the child's lead during daily activities being attentive and responsive to the child. As the opportunity arises, the clinician will place the symbol in proximity to the child and referent, while saying the word and touching the symbol to model indicating the symbol correspondence with the referent. The child may actually select the symbol to verify comprehension, which would be encouraged.

Preparation: The clinician will determine the nature of the symbols based on the child's level of development and the size, color, and contrast of the symbols based on the child's visual abilities. Although in this example, the child selected by pointing to or touching the symbol, the actual method of selection should be determined for each child based on his or her resources in motor control.

Other Clinical Considerations: Training may focus initially on only one symbol associated with a highly valued referent per context. For example, during snack time, the clinician may focus on modeling symbol referent association first for cookie, a favorite snack choice. However, this may be expanded. For example, next, the clinician may introduce the symbol for milk, after the child has demonstrated an understanding of that for cookie. Another context may be played where the first symbol to be trained is a highly valued toy. With mastery, symbol use in that context may also be expanded. In this fashion, the clinician helps the child develop a vocabulary based on what is salient for the child.

Codes: Td, PSc, Sc, Rc, Se, Pr, Ac, Hb, AAC.

Exemplar 7

Lizbeth Curme Stevens

Conceptually Define the Target Behavior: The child will be trained to communicate using a symbol.

Operationally Define the Treatment: The child will select a symbol to communicate his or her intent from an array of two symbols with 90 percent accuracy.

> **Environment**: Intervention should occur during naturally occurring routines. Training may be enhanced by increasing the child's need to communicate. Therefore, items that the child desires may be placed out of reach but within the child's line of vision (e.g., the child wants to color but the crayons are up on the shelf within sight but out of reach).

> **Materials**: Symbols that the child knows (correspond to referents) should be accessible and within reach of the child at all times (e.g., during playtime, book reading, mealtime, or snack time). Symbols may be affixed to items within the environment (e.g., symbols for favorite TV shows could be placed on or near the television; the symbol for cookie may be taped to the cookie jar). Alternatively, the symbols may be readily available in the form of communication boards, books, wallets, or on speech-generating devices. Targets for symbol usage are frequently desired activities or objects in the child's environment.

> **Stimulus Conditions**: The clinician will place desired objects out of the child's reach but within the child's visual field and wait for the child to request the items. If necessary, the clinician will verbally prompt the child to select the symbol representing the desired item. The symbol may be selected by either pointing to or touching the symbol. The child will be intrinsically reinforced by receiving the item requested.

Preparation: The clinician will determine the nature of the symbols based on the child's level of development and the size, color, and contrast of the symbols based on the child's visual abilities. While the child in the present example used pointing to and touching as a means of selecting, the actual method of selection should be determined for each child based on an evaluation of the child's level of motor control.

Other Clinical Considerations: To express needs using the symbols obviously assumes that the child already understands the correspondence between the symbol and the referent. The training has been addressed in exemplar 6, which may precede the current activity.

Codes: Td, PSc, Sc, Ex, Se, Pr, Ac, Hb, AAC.

Exemplar 8

Denise Kowalski

Conceptually Define the Target Behavior: The present progressive verb will be trained.

Operationally Define the Treatment: The child will verbally produce a subject + *is* + verbing sentence (e.g., *She is running*) in a picture description task when asked, *What is (he/she) doing?* with 90 percent accuracy.

> **Environment**: Intervention will occur in a quiet, well-lit room with the child and clinician sitting side-by-side at a child-sized table or even sitting on a carpeted floor as appropriate to handle the materials.
>
> **Materials**: The training items presented may vary along a continuum of abstraction from actual objects, such as dolls, to photographs to line drawings as appropriate to the needs of the child. In this example, pictures will be used.
>
> **Stimulus Conditions**: Initially, the clinician presents a picture depicting the present progressive verb and models the target response (subject + *is* + verbing). Then, the clinician presents another picture depicting the present progressive verb and asks the child to use the target response to verbally describe the picture. When the child says the target response correctly, the clinician provides reinforcement (praise, token, etc.) and presents the next stimulus item. If the child produces an incorrect response, the clinician presents a prompt in the form of a question (e.g., *What is she doing?* or *Who is jumping?*), whichever is appropriate to the child's error. If the child verbalizes the target response after the prompt, then the clinician provides reinforcement and presents the next stimulus item. If the child produces another incorrect response, a second prompt is provided appropriate to the child's error. If the child verbalizes the target response, reinforcement is provided and the clinician presents the next stimuli item. However, if the child verbalizes another incorrect response the clinician says (e.g., *That is not quite right. You should say, "She is jumping," but let's go on to the next one*).

Preparation: Before initiating treatment, the clinician should play with the child to makes sure that the child understands the vocabulary items to be used. The clinician should also determine that the child can understand the target form receptively and can imitate the target form.

Other Clinical Considerations: Initially, the stimulus items should only include single subject pictures. After mastery is achieved, the next logical step would be training the plural form, for example, *they are jumping*. Next, a maintenance experience would be appropriate in which the singular and plural forms are interspersed in the intervention.

Codes: PSc, Ex, Sn, Mr, Ac, CD.

Exemplar 9

Denise Kowalski

Conceptually Define the Target Behavior: The regular past tense verb will be trained.

Operationally Define the Treatment: The child will verbally produce a subject + verb*ed* + object noun phrase (e.g., *She washed her hands.*) in a picture description task when asked, *What did (he/she) do?* (or a similar question) with 90 percent accuracy.

Environment: Intervention will occur in a quiet, well-lit room with the child and clinician sitting side-by-side at a child-sized table or even sitting on a carpeted floor as appropriate to handling the materials.

Materials: The training items presented may vary along a continuum of abstraction from actual objects such as dolls to photos to line drawings as appropriate to the needs of the child. In this example, pictures will be used.

Stimulus Conditions: Initially, the clinician presents a picture depicting a regular past tense verb while stating a present progressive sentence form (e.g., *The girl is washing her hands*). The clinician then follows this statement by asking, *What did she do?* and models that she washed her hands. The clinician says, e.g., *Now it's your turn.* The clinician presents another picture depicting the present progressive verb and asks the child to use the target response to verbally tell what happened in the picture. When the child says the target response correctly, the clinician provides reinforcement (praise, token, etc.) and presents the next stimulus item. If the child produces an incorrect response, the clinician presents a prompt in the form of a question (e.g., *What did she do? Who washed their hands?* or *What did she wash?*), whichever is appropriate to the child's error. If the child verbalizes the target response after the prompt, then the clinician provides reinforcement and presents the next stimulus item. If the child produces another incorrect response, a second prompt is provided appropriate to the child's error. If the child verbalizes the target response, reinforcement is provided and the clinician presents the next stimuli item. However, if the child verbalizes another incorrect response, the clinician says something like,

That is not quite right, you should say, she washed her hands. But let's go on to the next one.

Preparation: Before initiating treatment, the clinician should play with the child to make sure that the child understands the vocabulary items to be used. The clinician should also determine that the child can understand the target form receptively and can imitate the target form. The child should also understand the temporal concepts of past and present.

Other Clinical Considerations: Initially, the stimulus items should only include single subject pictures. After mastery is achieved, a next logical step would be training the plural form; for example, *they washed their hands*. Next, a maintenance experience would be appropriate where present progressive and past tense forms are interspersed in the intervention.

Codes: PSc, Ex, Sn, Mr, Ac, CD.

Exemplar 10

Denise Kowalski

Conceptually Define the Target Behavior: The future tense verb will be trained.

Operationally Define the Treatment: The child will verbally produce a subject + will + verb (e.g., *She will eat*) in a picture description task when asked, *What will he/she do next?* or something similar, with 90 percent accuracy.

> **Environment**: Intervention will occur in a quiet, well-lit room with the child and clinician sitting side-by-side at a child-sized table or even sitting on a carpeted floor as appropriate to handling the materials.

> **Materials**: The training items presented may vary along a continuum of abstraction from actual objects such as dolls to photos to line drawings as appropriate to the needs of the child. In this example, pictures will be used.

> **Stimulus Conditions**: Initially, the clinician presents a two-picture sequence depicting two actions (e.g., getting dressed and eating breakfast). The clinician makes a statement describing the first picture (e.g., *The boy is getting dressed for school*). Then the clinician asks the question, *What will he do next?* or something similar, prompting the child to describe the second picture with the intended future tense target. If the child produces the correct response, the clinician provides reinforcement (verbal praise, token, etc.) and proceeds to the next stimuli. If the child produces an incorrect response, the clinician presents a prompt in the form of an incomplete model with emphasis on *will* (e.g., *The boy will* _____) prompting the child to provide the missing verb to complete the carrier phrase. Then, the clinician elicits the entire target response by repeating the question, *What will he do next?* using the same set of cards. If the child verbalizes the target response after the prompt, then the clinician provides reinforcement and presents the next stimulus item. If the child produces another incorrect response the clinician should say, *The boy will eat?* again emphasizing the word *will* followed by *What will the boy do?* If the child verbalizes the target response, reinforcement is provided and the clinician presents the next stimuli item.

However, if the child verbalizes another incorrect response, the clinician says something like, *That is not quite right. You should say, "He will eat breakfast," but let's go on to the next one.*

Preparation: Before initiating treatment, the clinician should play with the child to make sure that the child understands the vocabulary items to be used. The clinician should also determine that the child can understand the target form receptively and can imitate the target form. The child should also understand the temporal concepts of past, present, and future.

Other Clinical Considerations: This exemplar includes two pictures depicting verbs in a sequence. Initially, the stimulus should include two verb-sequence pictures. After mastery is achieved, the next logical step would be to provide only one picture and ask the child to self-formulate the next sentence in the sequence.

Codes: PSc, Ex, Sn, Mr, Ac, CD.

Exemplar 11

Ronald B. Hoodin

Conceptually Define the Target Behavior: The regular plural morpheme will be trained.

Operationally Define the Treatment: The child will point to the picture of more than one object (depicting the plural form) in an array of two pictures in response to a verbal instruction with 90 percent accuracy.

> **Environment**: Intervention will occur in a traditional, well-lit, quiet room with the child and clinician sitting on chairs opposite one another at a table.
>
> **Materials**: The pictures in the array of two will consist of one picture of two or more objects (depicting a plural) and one picture of a single object (depicting a singleton). The singleton picture serves as a foil. The order of presentation of the pictures from left to right should be randomized to avoid order effects, such as learning to always choose the picture on the right. The pictured objects will be common objects seen in the child's environment such as shoes, apples, and chairs.
>
> **Stimulus Conditions**: The clinician will present the array of two pictures plus a verbal instruction (e.g., *Point to the picture of the shoes or show me the shoes*) as discrete trials (one at a time with a brief pause between each presentation). When the child points to the correct picture, the clinician will provide positive verbal feedback (e.g., *that's right, good job*) and will move along to the next item. When the child points to the incorrect picture, the clinician will provide negative verbal feedback (e.g., *No, you pointed to the shoe, there is just one of them in that picture. I wanted you to point to shoes, emphasizing the plural marker with stress and modeling the correct response by pointing to the correct picture or something similar. Now let's redo that item.*). Then, the clinician will present the same item again. If the child is inaccurate the second time, the clinician will say something like (*No, it's this one while pointing to the correct one but let's move on.*) Repeated failure suggests that the child is not yet ready for the activity.

Preparation: Before administering the baseline, the clinician will informally play/interact with the child to ensure that the child can comply or participate with the structure of the activity. This may include understanding the vocabulary items and understanding what is expected of him or her by pointing to items as instructed.

Other Clinical Considerations: The target behavior, acquisition of the regular plural morpheme, may actually consist of more than one distinct behaviors: processing the /z/ allomorph as in the word <u>shoes</u>, processing the /s/ allomorph as in the word <u>mats</u>, and processing the /uz/ allomorph as in the word <u>matches</u>. If the response to training in the individual child does not include simultaneous acquisition of all relevant allomorphs, then each should be trained as distinct target behaviors. The issue may be relevant receptively or expressively.

After achieving mastery on this target behavior, the clinician may wish to take the following next logical step, selecting two target behaviors to train simultaneously (in the same activity but in separate discrete trials): pointing to the picture depicting plurals and pointing to the picture depicting the singletons.

Codes: PSc, Sc, Rc, Mr, Ac, CD.

Exemplar 12

Ronald B. Hoodin

Conceptually Define the Target Behavior: The use of appropriate adjectives with count nouns and mass nouns will be trained.

Operationally Define the Treatment: The student will indicate whether sentences are correct or incorrect with regard to adjective-count noun and adjective-mass noun combinations with 90 percent accuracy.

Environment: Intervention will occur in a classroom with the teacher projecting sentences on a screen for the class to view.

Materials: The projected sentences will include those with adjective-count noun combinations that are correct (e.g., *I see three dogs*) and incorrect (e.g., *I want more dog*). In addition, the projected sentences will include adjective–mass noun combinations that are correct (e.g., *I want some steak*) and incorrect (e.g., *I want three water*). Count nouns get their name from the fact that a number can modify them. Conversely, a number cannot be used to modify a mass noun. However, mass nouns may be partitioned and then modified with numbers (e.g., *I want three pieces of steak* or *I want two teaspoons of sugar*).

Stimulus Conditions: The teacher projects a randomly ordered sentence on the screen and reads the sentence to the class. The students repeat the sentence in unison. Then the students are asked whether the sentence is correct or incorrect. When the students are right, the teacher provides positive feedback (e.g., that's right, good) and continues with the next sentence. When the students are wrong, the teacher points out the error based on the rule for using adjectives with count and mass nouns (described under materials) and continues with the next sentence.

Preparation: This activity draws on both the students' metalinguistic and reading skills. The ability to read is helpful here but not actually necessary because the sentence is both written and spoken. The students repeat the sentence to enhance its presence.

Other Clinical Considerations: After completing this activity, the teacher may wish to consider assigning a writing activity, which requires the use of adjectives with both count and mass nouns.

Codes: PSc, Sc, Rc, Sn, Mr, Ac, CD, AL.

Exemplar 13

Ronald B. Hoodin

Conceptually Define the Target Behavior: Appropriate eye contact during conversation will be trained.

Operationally Define the Treatment: The student will use appropriate eye contact in dyadic communication with the clinician with 90 percent accuracy. Appropriate eye contact means that the student avoids locking into the clinicians' eyes. Instead, eye contact occurs briefly with the onset of a conversational turn, at the termination of a conversational turn and intermittently during the turn.

> **Environment**: Intervention will occur in a well-lit, quiet room with the clinician and student sitting adjacent to one another on chairs.

> **Materials**: The clinician has a list of topics that the student would be able to sustain in a conversation for several conversational turns.

> **Stimulus Conditions**: The student and clinician engage in a conversation in a dyad. The clinician models appropriate eye contact and explains what he or she is doing. Then, the student imitates the model. As the student does so, the clinician provides feedback, prompts, and encouragement. As the student acquires the target behavior, the models and prompts are faded.

Preparation: Before training is initiated, the clinician interviews the students and perhaps others such as parents, teachers, and peers to develop a list of interests or topics that the student would be able to sustain for several turns in the conversations.

Other Clinical Considerations: This intervention procedure is derived from and extends the notion of script training, which was described in Chapter 6. After training this target behavior, it would be logical to provide an activity to facilitate generalization. See exemplar 14.

Codes: PSc, Sc, Pr, Ac, Hb.

Exemplar 14

Ronald B. Hoodin

Conceptually Define the Target Behavior: Appropriate eye contact during conversation will be trained at the level of generalization.

Operationally Define the Treatment: The clinician will teach the student the rule for maintaining appropriate eye contact during conversations and rely on the student's self-management skills to implement the skill in untrained communicative environments. The rule is that the student avoids locking onto someone's gaze. Instead, the student makes brief eye contact at the initiation of a conversational turn, at the termination of a conversational turn, and intermittently during the conversational turn.

> **Environment**: The student goes out to his or her typical communicative environments (e.g., home, recess, lunchroom, classroom, gym class) and implements the generalization procedure.
>
> **Materials**: The student has the rule written down and reads it from time to time.
>
> **Stimulus Conditions**: The clinician reviews the rule for appropriate eye contact during conversations with the student and asks the student to go out into his or her various communicative environments and implement the rule. The student periodically returns to be interviewed by the clinician who provides feedback, insights, and encouragements.

Preparation: Before participating in this generalization procedure, the student would have completed the acquisition of the target behavior that was addressed in exemplar 13.

Other Clinical Considerations: This generalization procedure reflects a notion called mediated generalization, which is reviewed in Chapter 6.

Codes: PSc, Sc, Pr, Gn, Hb.

Exemplar 15

Ana Claudia Harten

Conceptually Define the Target Behavior: The prepositions *on*, *in*, *under*, and *over* will be trained.

Operationally Define the Treatment: The child will follow and express one-step commands involving the locative prepositions with 90 percent accuracy.

> **Environment**: This intervention can take place in different settings. It can occur in a traditional individual therapy room, in a group therapy room, or at a school recreation room/gym or playground.
>
> **Materials**: The objects/toys selected for this activity should be common objects/toys seen in the child's school or home environment (e.g., a doll to be placed in a dollhouse, a ball to be placed under a table). For culturally and linguistically diverse (CLD) children, the clinician should interview the children's parents to find out what kinds of objects/toys are common in their home environment.
>
> **Stimulus Conditions**: The clinician and the child will play the Simon Says game. The game will incorporate one-step commands involving placement of objects/toys in specific locations determined by the game Simon Says. The clinician says something like, "Simon says put the doll in the house," and the child is supposed to do so. However, if the clinician neglects to say, "Simon says" and just says, "put the doll in the house," then the child is supposed to not respond.
>
> When the child places the object correctly, the clinician provides positive verbal feedback (e.g., *good job*) and gives tokens for correct responses that can be traded for a prize at the end of the session. If the child places the object/toy incorrectly, the clinician corrects the response, emphasizing the preposition with stress and modeling the correct placement of the object/toy (e.g., *No, you placed the doll <u>on</u> the house. I asked you to place the doll <u>in</u> the house, like this. You see, the doll is <u>in</u> the house now. Place the doll <u>in</u> the house again.*). The clinician starts the game and when the child masters the skill receptively, he/she can take turns being the one saying the commands while the clinician executes them. The clinician should occasionally

make an incorrect execution, requiring the child to identify correct and incorrect responses.

Preparation: Before beginning this activity, the clinician needs to make sure that the child is familiar with the objects/toys and understands what is expected from him or her. For the child who is not familiar with the Simon Says game, the clinician needs to demonstrate the game and model some responses for the child before beginning the activity.

Other Clinical Considerations: For bilingual children, it would be more beneficial to conduct this activity in both languages, that is, in English and in the child's first language. If the clinician is bilingual or if an interpreter or volunteer is available, the intervention should be conducted in both languages, which could be done in blocks of sessions for each language, incorporating the use of both languages at a time whenever necessary. If the clinician is unable to provide intervention in the child's first language, the parents/siblings should be trained to do the same kind of activity (or similar activities targeting the same goal) at home using the child's first language.

Codes: PSc, Sc, Rc, Ex, Se, Ac, CD, Mc.

Exemplar 16

Ronald B. Hoodin

Conceptually Define the Target Behavior: The expressive use of noun phrases will be expanded.

Operationally Define the Treatment: The students will say a sentence containing an expanded noun phrase (e.g., *She is wearing a blue striped blouse*) with 90 percent accuracy.

> **Environment**: Intervention will occur in a well-lit, quiet room with several students and the clinician sitting facing one another at a table.
>
> **Materials**: Pictures taken from catalogs that sell clothing will serve as the stimulus items.
>
> **Stimulus Conditions**: The clinician explains that the students are required to describe what the person is wearing using a sentence containing words for an article + color + pattern + noun (e.g., *He is wearing a red striped shirt*). The clinician shows the picture and asks the question (e.g., *What is he/she wearing?*) to elicit responding. When the students provide an accurate sentence, positive feedback is provided (e.g., *that's right, good*), and the next stimulus item is presented. However, when a deficient response is elicited, the clinician provides appropriate prompts (e.g., *What was the color?*).

Preparation: The clinician should make sure that each student knows the vocabulary used in the activity and can repeat the sentences used.

Other Clinical Considerations: After mastering the target behavior with clothing, a logical next step would be to expand the noun phrase describing other nouns in the object position (e.g., *She sat on a large green sofa*). At some point, the clinician may want to focus on expanding the noun phrase in the subject position (e.g., *The large black dog jumped over the fence*). Of course, eventually the noun phrases in both the object and subject position may be expanded (e.g., *The large black dog broke the small yellow vase*).

Codes: PSc, Sc, Ex, Sn, Mr, Ac, CD.

Exemplar 17

Linda J. Polter

Conceptually Define the Target Behavior: The gerund form as a direct object will be trained.

Operationally Define the Treatment: The child will verbally produce a sentence containing the gerund form as a direct object (e.g., *I like swimming*) when given a picture training stimulus item with 100 percent accuracy.

> **Environment**: The intervention will occur in a traditional, well-lit, quiet room with the child and teacher sitting on chairs at a table.
>
> **Materials**: The teacher will have several carrier phrases (e.g., *I like*) on a white board that serve as prompts and several training stimulus pictures that illustrate simple action verbs with which the child would be familiar (e.g., *swimming, running, playing*).
>
> **Stimulus Conditions**: The teacher will explain to the child that he or she is expected to verbally produce sentences containing the gerund as a direct object. The teacher will model using the carrier phrase prompt (e.g., *I like*), show a picture stimulus, and then finish the sentence (e.g., *I like swimming*). The teacher will then elicit the target form using the carrier phrases as prompts and pictures as training stimuli. When the child says the sentence correctly, the teacher will provide positive verbal feedback (e.g., *good job, that's a good sentence*) and will give the child another picture stimulus. If the child does not say the sentence correctly, the teacher will model the correct sentence and then have the child repeat the sentence. The teacher will then give the child another picture stimulus.

Preparation: Before beginning this task, the teacher would interact with the child to ensure that the child understands the language form receptively, understands the task, and can repeat the sentence. The child should also understand the vocabulary used in the prompts and training stimulus pictures.

Other Clinical Considerations: This strategy uses a teaching technique called "patterning" that was developed at St. Joseph Institute for the Deaf by Sister Jeanne d'Arc (Buckler, 1967). Patterning is a language approach designed to teach and reinforce complex language

forms by example rather than by explanation. As this activity progresses, the child will develop a cadre of sentences using this language
structure. As a review, the teacher points to a picture and the child says
the entire sentence.

Codes: Sc, Ex, Sn, Mr, Ac, CD, AL.

Reference

Buckler, M. S., Sr. (1967). *Expanding language through patterning*. Paper presented at the Fifth Congress of the World Federation of the Deaf, Warsaw,
Poland.

Exemplar 18

Linda J. Polter

Conceptually Define the Target Behavior: The infinitive form as a direct object will be trained.

Operationally Define the Treatment: The child will verbally produce a sentence containing the infinitive form as a direct object (e.g., *I like to swim*) when given a picture training stimulus item with 100 percent accuracy.

> **Environment**: The intervention will occur in a traditional, well-lit, quiet room with the child and teacher sitting on chairs at a table.
>
> **Materials**: The teacher will have several carrier phrases (e.g., *I like*) on a white board, which serve as prompts and several training stimulus pictures that illustrate simple action verbs with which the child would be familiar (e.g., *to swim, to run, to play*).
>
> **Stimulus Conditions**: The teacher will explain to the child that he or she is expected to verbally produce sentences containing the infinitive as a direct object. The teacher will model using the carrier phrase prompt (e.g., *I like*), show a picture stimulus, and then finish the sentence (e.g., *I like to swim*). Then the teacher will elicit the target form using the carrier phrases as prompts and pictures as training stimuli. When the child says the sentence correctly, the teacher will provide positive verbal feedback (e.g., *good job, that's a good sentence*) and will give the child another picture stimulus. If the child does not say the sentence correctly, the teacher will model the correct sentence and then have the child repeat the sentence. The teacher will then give the child another picture stimulus.

Preparation: Before beginning this task, the teacher would interact with the child to ensure that the child understands the language form receptively, understands the task, and can repeat the sentence. The child should also understand the vocabulary used in the prompts and training stimulus pictures.

Other Clinical Considerations: This strategy uses a teaching technique called "patterning" that was developed at St. Joseph Institute for the Deaf by Sister Jeanne d'Arc (Buckler, 1967). Patterning is a language approach designed to teach and reinforce complex language forms by example rather than by explanation. As this activity progresses, the child will develop a cadre of sentences using this language structure. As a review, the teacher points to a picture and the child says the entire sentence.

Codes: Sc, Ex, Sn, Mr, Ac, CD, AL.

Reference

Buckler, M. S., Sr. (1967). *Expanding language through patterning*. Paper presented at the Fifth Congress of the World Federation of the Deaf, Warsaw, Poland.

Exemplar 19
Linda J. Polter

Conceptually Define the Target Behavior: The gerund form as a direct object will be generalized.

Operationally Define the Treatment: The children will verbally produce sentences containing the gerund form as a direct object (e.g., *I like swimming*) when given a picture training stimulus item with 100 percent accuracy.

> **Environment**: The intervention will occur in a traditional, well-lit, quiet room with the children and teacher sitting in a small group (three to six children) around a table.
>
> **Materials**: The teacher will have several carrier phrases (e.g., *I like*) on a white board that serve as prompts and several training stimulus pictures that illustrate simple action verbs with which the children would be familiar (e.g., *swimming, running, playing*).
>
> **Stimulus Conditions**: The teacher will explain to the children that they are expected to produce sentences containing the gerund as a direct object. The teacher will model using the carrier phrase prompt (e.g., *I like*), show a picture stimulus, and then finish the sentence (e.g., *I like swimming*). The teacher will then elicit the target form using the carrier phrases as prompts and pictures as training stimuli. When a child says the sentence correctly, the teacher will provide positive verbal feedback (e.g., *good job, that's a good sentence*) and will give the child another picture stimulus. If the child does not say the sentence correctly, the teacher will model the correct sentence and then have the child repeat the sentence. The teacher will then give the child another picture stimulus.

Preparation: Each child would have attended individual sessions with the teacher to teach this language form at the acquisition level (see exemplar 17) before participating in this generalization intervention.

Other Clinical Considerations: This strategy uses a teaching technique called "patterning" that was developed at St. Joseph Institute for the Deaf by Sister Jeanne d'Arc (Buckler, 1967). Patterning is a language approach designed to teach and reinforce complex language forms by example rather than by explanation. As this activity progresses, the children will develop a cadre of sentences using this language structure. As a review, the teacher points to a picture and the child says the entire sentence.

Codes: Sc, Ex, Sn, Mr, Gn, CD, AL.

Reference

Buckler, M. S., Sr. (1967). *Expanding language through patterning*. Paper presented at the Fifth Congress of the World Federation of the Deaf, Warsaw, Poland.

Exemplar 20
Linda J. Polter

Conceptually Define the Target Behavior: The infinitive form as a direct object will be generalized.

Operationally Define the Treatment: The children will verbally produce sentences containing the infinitive form as a direct object (e.g., *I like to swim*) when given a picture training stimulus item with 100 percent accuracy.

> **Environment**: The intervention will occur in a traditional, well-lit, quiet room with the children and teacher sitting in a small group (three to six children) around a table.

> **Materials**: The teacher will have several carrier phrases (e.g., *I like*) on a white board that serve as prompts and several training stimulus pictures that illustrate simple action verbs with which the children would be familiar (e.g., *to swim, to run, to play*).

> **Stimulus conditions**: The teacher will explain to the children that they are expected to produce sentences containing the infinitive as a direct object. The teacher will model using the carrier phrase prompt (e.g., *I like*), show a picture stimulus, and then finish the sentence (e.g., *I like to swim*). The teacher will then elicit the target form using the carrier phrases as prompts and pictures as training stimuli. When a child says the sentence correctly, the teacher will provide positive verbal feedback (e.g., *good job, that's a good sentence*) and will give the child another picture stimulus. If the child does not say the sentence correctly, the teacher will model the correct sentence and then have the child repeat the sentence. The teacher will then give the child another picture stimulus.

Preparation: Each child would have attended individual sessions with the teacher to teach this language form at the acquisition level (see exemplar 18) before participating in this generalization intervention.

Other Clinical Considerations: This strategy uses a teaching technique called "patterning" that was developed at St. Joseph Institute for the Deaf by Sister Jeanne d'Arc (Buckler, 1967). Patterning is a language approach designed to teach and reinforce complex language forms by example rather than by explanation. As this activity progresses, the children will develop a cadre of sentences using this language structure. As a review, the teacher points to a picture and the child says the entire sentence.

Codes: Sc, Ex, Sn, Mr, Gn, CD, AL.

Reference

Buckler, M. S., Sr. (1967). *Expanding language through patterning*. Paper presented at the Fifth Congress of the World Federation of the Deaf, Warsaw, Poland.

Exemplar 21

Ronald B. Hoodin

Conceptually Define the Target Behavior: Increase the student's metalinguistic awareness of the nature of metaphors in preparation for teaching the student to explain metaphors. (Recall that a metaphor describes one referent in terms of another.)

Operationally Define the Treatment: The child will respond to multiple choice fill-ins, riddles, and explicit sentences with 90 percent accuracy to demonstrate his or her understanding of the metaphor.

Environment: Intervention will occur in a quiet room with the clinician and student sitting on chairs opposite one another at a table.

Materials: Stimulus items should be developed individually for each metaphor and include multiple choice fill-ins (e.g., *The speed boat _____.* where (a) *traveled fast*, is literal and (b) *was a rocket*, is metaphorical.), riddles (e.g., *What spins like a top but does so on the ice?* The answer is a *figure skater*), and sentences that make the similarity between the two referents explicit (e.g., *A giraffe is tall like a flagpole*).

Stimulus Conditions: The clinician explains that metaphors describe one referent in terms of another (e.g., *My daughter is a jewel*). To understand this sentence, the listener rejects the literal message, which is absurd yet marks the presence of the metaphor and simultaneously provides clues to the intended message. That is, a jewel is precious so the underlying message is that my daughter is precious. Next, the clinician increases the student's metalinguistic awareness of the nature of the metaphor by using the aforementioned stimulus items.

Preparation: No specific preparation is required. However, the child would be expected to possess sufficient cognitive resources to participate in the task. As such, the child would likely be school age.

Other Clinical Considerations: This intervention is based on Wallach and Miller (1988). It serves to prepare the child for the next logical step, explaining metaphors in exemplar 22.

Codes: Sc, Rc, Se, Ac, CD, AL.

Reference

Wallach, G. P., & Miller, L. (1988). *Language intervention and academic success.* San Diego, CA: College Hill Press.

Exemplar 22
Ronald B. Hoodin

Conceptually Define the Target Behavior: Identifying and explaining metaphors will be trained.

Operationally Define the Treatment: The student will identify the presence of a metaphor and then explain it with 90 percent accuracy.

> **Environment**: Intervention will occur in a quiet room with the student and clinician sitting on chairs opposite one another at a table.
>
> **Materials**: The clinician will use a series of metaphors in a monologue that serves as the stimulus items.
>
> **Stimulus Conditions**: The clinician verbally presents a monologue that includes a series of metaphors. The student identifies the presence of each metaphor based on its absurd literal interpretation. If the student is correct in identifying the metaphor, then positive feedback is provided and the student is asked to explain the intended or metaphoric message. If the student does not correctly identify the metaphor, the clinician uses prompts to help the student make an accurate identification (e.g., *Is a daughter really a jewel? Is a speed boat really a rocket? Is a giraffe really a flagpole?*).
>
> Once the student accurately identifies the metaphor (e.g., *My daughter is a jewel. The speed boat is a rocket. A giraffe is a flagpole living at the zoo.*), the student is asked to explain the metaphor. If the student is accurate in his or her explanation, the clinician provides positive feedback and encouragement and goes on with the monologue. However, if the student is inaccurate, the clinician provides prompts to help the student make an accurate interpretation (e.g., *A jewel is precious what is being said about my daughter? A rocket is really fast, so what is being said about the speed boat? A flagpole is really tall, so what is being said about the giraffe?*).

Preparation: Beforehand, the student should complete exemplar 21, which teaches metalinguistic awareness of metaphors.

Other Clinical Considerations: This intervention is based on Wallach and Miller (1988).

Codes: Sc, Rc, Ex, Se. Ac, CD, LA.

Reference

Wallach, G. P., & Miller, L. (1988). *Language intervention and academic success.* San Diego, CA: College Hill Press.

Exemplar 23

Ronald B. Hoodin

Conceptually Define the Target Behavior: Telling personal narratives will be trained.

Operationally Define the Treatment: The student will tell a personal narrative characterized by narrative coherence with 90 percent accuracy. Narrative coherence will include (1) topic maintenance, whether all utterances relate to the topic; (2) event sequencing, whether the events are logically sequenced; (3) informativeness, whether there is sufficient detail; (4) referencing, whether there is adequate identification of individuals, locations, features; (5) conjunctive cohesion, whether the words (e.g., *then, because, so, but*) link the events together; and (6) fluency, whether there is sufficient momentum to the spoken presentation.

> **Environment**: Intervention will take place in a quiet, well-lit room with the student and clinician sitting adjacent to one another at a table.

> **Materials:** The student draws the story to be told using stick-figure drawings. These drawings serve as prompts as the student tells the story.

> **Stimulus Conditions**: The clinician first models drawing a personal story using stick-figure drawings and then telling the story while using stick-figure drawings as prompts. Then, the student is asked to draw his or her own personal story and do the same. During the student's presentation, the clinician uses *wh-* questions (e.g., *who, what, where, when, how*) to prompt the student. However, to avoid overwhelming the student, the clinician selects only one dimension at a time to focus on (e.g., topic maintenance). The clinician first provides prompts regarding the first three dimensions, which are more basic before the last three dimensions.

Preparation: Beforehand, the clinician explains the notion of telling personal narratives and underscores its importance.

Other Clinical Considerations: This clinical procedure uses the Narrative Assessment Profile (NAP) developed by McCabe and Bliss (2003). It also reflects ideas for implementing training, which they developed. The clinician may review training students to tell personal narratives as in Chapter 6. The next logical step would be to facilitate generalization of the target behavior to the classroom environment. See exemplar 24.

Codes: Sc, Ex, Pr, Ac, Hb, AL.

Reference

McCabe, A., & Bliss, L. S. (2003). *Patterns of narrative discourse: A multicultural, life span approach*. Boston, MA: Pearson Education.

Exemplar 24

Ronald B. Hoodin

Conceptually Define the Target Behavior: Telling personal narratives will be trained at the level of generalization.

Operationally Define the Treatment: The student will tell a personal narrative characterized by narrative coherence with 90 percent accuracy. Narrative coherence will include (1) topic maintenance, whether all utterances relate to the topic; (2) event sequencing, whether the events are logically sequenced; (3) informativeness, whether there is sufficient detail; (4) referencing, whether there is adequate identification of individuals, locations, features; (5) conjunctive cohesion, whether the words (e.g., *then, because, so, but*, etc.) link the events together; and (6) fluency, whether there is sufficient momentum to the spoken presentation.

> **Environment**: Intervention will take place in a traditional classroom where the student comes to the front of the classroom and tells the story to the classmates.
>
> **Materials**: The student draws the story to be told using stick-figure drawings. These drawings serve as prompts as the student tells the story.
>
> **Stimulus Conditions**: The student tells the story to classmates who will also be telling their stories subsequently. The classmates are an attentive, supportive audience. At the end of the presentation, the classmates fill out a card providing feedback to the presenter regarding his or her performance along the six dimensions of narrative coherence. After reading and digesting the feedback, the student meets with the clinician to discuss the presentation and the feedback, as well as opportunities for continued improvement.

Preparation: All of the members of the class will have completed exemplar 23, where each received training in telling personal narratives on the level of acquisition. All of the students will be familiar with the six dimensions of narrative cohesion. The entire class will be instructed by the clinician on evaluating each of the six dimensions as good, neutral, or needs improvement so that they can provide feedback. The students will be instructed regarding the importance of providing each presenter with a supportive audience, which empowers the student to tell a good story.

Other Clinical Considerations: Many of the ideas used in this training procedure, as well as the Narrative Assessment Profile (NAP), were derived from McCabe and Bliss (2003).

Codes: Sc, Ex, Pr, Gn, Hb, AL.

Reference

McCabe, A., & Bliss, L. S. (2003). *Patterns of narrative discourse: A multicultural, life span approach*. Boston, MA: Pearson Education.

Exemplar 25

Brenda Doster

Conceptually Define the Target Behavior: Metalinguistic awareness of idioms will be trained at level I. For this exemplar, training the idiom *lend a hand* will serve as an example.

Operationally Define the Treatment: The students will point to a picture depicting the figurative interpretation of the idiom in an array of two pictures where the foil depicts the literal interpretation in response to a verbal instruction with 90 percent accuracy.

Environment: Intervention will occur in an elementary classroom with up to about seven students. The students and teacher will be seated in chairs positioned around a table.

Materials: Besides the table and chairs, there will be books and markers to be used as props. The teacher will use pairs of pictures with each idiom; one will depict a figurative representation of the idiom, whereas the other will depict a literal interpretation of it. The order of presentation of the pictures from left to right should be randomized to avoid teaching the child to choose the picture based on position.

Stimulus Conditions: The teacher begins by engaging the students in several skits designed to teach the figurative interpretation of the idiom *lend a hand*. In the first skit, the teacher has the books strewn haphazardly across the table and says something like, *Can you lend me a hand and put the books on the shelf?* Once the students help put the books away, the teacher says something like, *Thanks for lending me a hand with the books.*

In the second skit, the chairs are not aligned around the table and the teacher says something like, *Would you lend a hand and place the chairs neatly around the table?* After the students help reposition the chairs, the teacher says something like, *Thanks for lending a hand with the chairs.*

In the third skit, the teacher spills a box of markers that scatter on the floor and says something like, *Would you lend a hand and help pick up the markers?* After the students help gathering the markers the teacher says something like, *Thanks for lending a hand with the markers.*

After teaching the figurative interpretation of the idiom in the skits, the teacher determines mastery by presenting two pictures depicting the target idiom: one literally and one figuratively. The students are asked to select the picture that depicts *lend me a hand washing the car*. Ten idioms are taught, and the teacher presents the pairs of pictures in random order to determine whether criterion has been met.

Preparation: The teacher makes sure that the students understand the vocabulary words used in the training task, as well as making sure that the students understand what is required of them in the activity.

Other Clinical Considerations: To facilitate generalization of meta-linguistic awareness of the trained idioms to nontrained contexts, the teacher may use the idioms throughout the day, recruit parents and others to do the same, and post the idioms in conspicuous places such as the bulletin board. After the student completes level I training, he or she is ready for level II training (exemplar 26).

Codes: Sc, Rc, Se, Ac, Hb, AL.

Exemplar 26

Brenda Doster

Conceptually Define the Target Behavior: Metalinguistic awareness of idioms will be trained at level II. For this exemplar, training the idiom *lend a hand* will serve as an example.

Operationally Define the Treatment: The students will point to a picture depicting the figurative interpretation of the idiom in an array of two pictures in which the foil depicts the literal interpretation in response to a verbal instruction with 90 percent accuracy.

Environment: Intervention will occur in an elementary classroom with up to about seven students. The students and teacher will be seated in chairs positioned around a table.

Materials: The teacher will use pairs of pictures with each idiom; one will depict a figurative representation of the idiom, whereas the other will depict a literal interpretation of it. The order of presentation of the pictures from left to right should be randomized to avoid having the child learn to choose the picture based on its position. The pictures will depict helping situations to reinforce the idiom *lend a hand*.

Stimulus Conditions: The clinician will present the array of two pictures (one indicating an individual helping someone and the other showing a person's hand actually removed from his or her wrist) plus a verbal instruction (e.g., *point to lend a hand*) as discrete trials (one at a time with a brief pause between each presentation). When the student points to the correct picture, the teacher will provide positive verbal feedback (e.g., *that's right, good job*) and will move along to the next item. When the student points to the incorrect picture, the teacher will provide negative verbal feedback (e.g., *No, you pointed to the picture of someone giving someone a hand. Can we really remove our hand to give to someone? Now let's redo that item.*). Then, the teacher will present the same item again. If the student is inaccurate the second time, the teacher will say something like, "No, it's this one [while pointing to the correct one], but let's move on." Repeated failure suggests that the child is not yet ready for the activity.

Preparation: The student should complete exemplar 25 before participating in exemplar 26. The teacher should also ensure that the student understands the vocabulary and what is expected of him or her in the activity.

Other Clinical Considerations: To facilitate generalization of meta-linguistic awareness of the trained idioms to nontrained contexts, the teacher should continue to use the idioms throughout the day when appropriate.

Codes: Sc, Rc, Se, Ac, CD, AL.

Exemplar 27
Ana Claudia Harten

Conceptually Define the Target Behavior: Coherence in oral narratives involving curriculum-based contents will be trained.

Operationally Define the Treatment: The child will arrange a set of six pictures into a suitable chronological sequence and use them as prompts to tell a coherent narrative with 90 percent accuracy.

Environment: This intervention can occur in a traditional individual therapy room or in a group therapy room (in the case of a small-group session).

Materials: Each set of six pictures should depict a specific topic, with a clear beginning, middle, and end. The pictures should be given to the child in a random order to avoid influencing the child. The topics should reflect curriculum-based content, which would support the child's educational needs. This is particularly relevant for CLD children and others who are at risk educationally. For example, the clinician can take advantage of an upcoming class presentation and incorporate the presentation topic in this activity (e.g., caterpillar life cycle; animal evolution). The activity would help the child to participate successfully in the class presentation.

Another possibility would be the clinician collaborating with the teacher and selecting a grade-level book that is related to the child's culture to be read and discussed in class. The clinician could use the book to generate the topic (or topics) for the pictures. The activity would be used to help the child to participate in the class discussion. By doing that, the teacher and the clinician would not only be using a culturally appropriate topic and valuing the child's culture, but they would also be providing a chance for the bilingual child to use the vocabulary in his or her first language to bridge the vocabulary items into English.

Stimulus Conditions: The clinician will present a set of six pictures in a randomized order to the child and request that the child arrange the pictures in a chronological order. After arranging the pictures, the child is requested to tell a narrative describing the pictures (e.g., *These pictures are telling a story about caterpillars' life cycle that you learned in class. I want you to put these pictures in order, making* *sure that the story has a beginning, middle, and end. After you arrange the pictures, I want you to tell me the story.*). If the child arranges the pictures correctly and presents a coherent narrative with beginning, middle, and end, the clinician will provide positive verbal feedback (e.g., *good job*) and will move along to the next set of pictures. If the child arranges the pictures incorrectly or presents an incoherent narrative (e.g., lacking appropriate conjunctions, inappropriate sequencing, or missing important information), the clinician corrects the child and provides an appropriate model, stressing the main parts of the arrangement or narrative.

Preparation: Before beginning this activity, the clinician needs to make sure that the child understands what is expected from him or her. In addition, the clinician needs to make sure that the child is familiar with the topic. In case of using a curriculum-based content, the clinician can take the opportunity to review the topic with the child prior to the activity.

Other Clinical Considerations: As the child progresses, the number of pictures in the set can be increased, and the relationship between the components in the pictures can become more complex. In addition, whenever the clinician has an opportunity, he or she should link oral and written language as much as possible in various activities to promote school success, especially when working with CLD children. In the case of the present activity, besides the oral narrative, the clinician can easily incorporate in this activity the request for the child to create a written text describing the story displayed by the pictures.

For bilingual children, it would be more beneficial to conduct this activity in both languages, that is, in English and in the child's first language, which could be done in blocks of sessions for each language. If, for some reason, the clinician is unable to provide intervention in the child's first language, the parents/siblings should be trained to do the same kind of activity at home using the child's first language.

Codes: Sc, Rc, Ex, Se, Sn, Mr, Pr, Ac, CD, Mc, AL.

Exemplar 28
Ronald B. Hoodin

Conceptually Define the Target Behavior: The auxiliary verbs *would*, *should*, and *could* will be trained receptively.

Operationally Define the Treatment: The students will identify the correct written sentence using *would*, *should*, or *could* from an array of three sentences to characterize a story with 90 percent accuracy.

> **Environment**: Intervention will occur in a traditional classroom with the teacher at the front of the class.
>
> **Materials**: The teacher tells a brief story that involves conditions that could be described with the auxiliary verbs *would*, *could*, or *should*. Three written sentences are presented on an overhead associated with each story. One contains the word *would*; another contains the word *should*, and the third contains the word *could*. One sentence is correct while the other two serve as foils. Order of presentation is randomized to avoid order effects in learning.
>
> **Stimulus Conditions**: The teacher explains that she or he is teaching the meaning of the terms *would*, *should*, and *could*. The teacher indicates that *would* is used when the situation depends on something else (e.g., *Jennifer would take the job if it were offered*). The term *should* is used either when it is a good idea or because it is the right thing to do (e.g., *Jennifer should wear the heavy coat because it's cold* or *Jennifer should return the money that she found*). *Could* is used to indicate what is possible (e.g., *Jennifer could run the 6-minute mile*).
>
> Next, the teacher tells a brief story that could be depicted using the target forms. After telling the story, the teacher projects the three sentences from the overhead and asks the class which is the correct sentence and the rationale for the decision. If the students select the correct sentence, the teacher provides positive feedback (e.g., *that's right, good*) and continues on with the next story. When the students do not make the correct selection, the teacher provides prompts based on the distinctive meanings of the terms (e.g., *Did the story relate to what is possible?*).

Preparation: The teacher makes sure that the students have both meta-linguistic and reading skills to participate in the activity.

Other Clinical Considerations: The teacher may wish to follow up with a writing assignment that uses the terms.

Codes: Sc, Rc, Se, Sn, Mr, Ac, CD, AL.

Exemplar 29
Bill Cupples

Conceptually Define the Target Behavior: Students will learn the organization of expository text to improve comprehension.

Operationally Define the Treatment: The student will describe the organization of a portion of a chapter of the text that contains compare and contrast statements.

> **Environment**: Intervention will take place in a group setting of middle-school students with language impairments.
>
> **Materials**: The science textbook for the appropriate grade level.
>
> **Stimulus Condition**: The clinician will instruct the group to open their science text to a portion of a chapter that compares and contrasts various plant groups.
>
> **Preparation**: The clinician presents a diagram on a flip chart that shows the group how to compare and contrast concepts they will read in the text. The diagram organizes the information from topic to subtopics and instructs the students to describe what is alike and what is different.

Topic:

      Subtopic:

            Alike:

            Different:

      Subtopic:

            Alike:

            Different:

      Subtopic:

            Alike:

            Different:

The group reads the chapter and determines the topics, the labels of the various plant groups described in the chapter. After they have described the topics, they list the subtopics, the descriptions of the plant groups. After describing the plant groups, they determine what is similar and what is different about the plant groups. They determine the distinguishing features of the various plant groups.

Other Clinical Considerations: The organization of the comparing and contrasting was derived from Merritt and Culatta (1998).

Codes: Sc, Rc, Ex, Se, Pr, Hb, AL.

Reference

Merritt, D., & Cullatta, B. (1998). *Language intervention in the classroom*. San Diego, CA: Singular Publishing Group.

Exemplar 30
Bill Cupples

Conceptually Define the Target Behavior: Using story grammars to tell a story will be trained.

Operationally Define the Treatment: The students will write a story in a logical, sequential fashion, reflecting story grammar with the following elements: setting, initiating event or problem, internal response of the character(s), the plan of the character(s) in response to the event, the attempt of the character(s) to carry out the plan, the consequence of the attempt, and the character(s) reaction to the consequence. The story should contain appropriate syntax and be in full sentences.

> **Environment**: Intervention will take place in a group setting with five middle school students with language impairments.
>
> **Materials**: Pictures of school-aged children in a parklike setting and of a lost child. A flip chart with the story grammar elements listed will set on an easel.
>
> **Stimulus Condition**: The clinician will present a situation to the group using the pictures. The group will be instructed to construct a story given the situation described by the clinician. They will be instructed to use all seven elements of the story grammar they have learned in previous sessions. As the group constructs the story using the elements of story grammar as prompts, one member will write the story on the flip chart. After the story is written, the clinician will ask the group to evaluate their story based on their use of the story grammar elements.

Preparation: The clinician will make sure that the students understand the task and the elements of story grammar before participating in the activity.

Other Clinical Considerations: The group constructed the following story:

Setting: Jim, Alexis, Tom, and Ashley were hanging out in the park one day deciding what they would do next.

Initiating event: Alexis noticed a crying 5-year-old boy standing alone by a bench.

Internal response: Alexis is upset by the child, and tells the others what she sees. Jim and Tom say that they shouldn't get involved; they are sure that the boy will find his mother or father. Ashley says they should go over to the child to ask what's wrong with him.

Plan of the characters: Alexis and Ashley convince the boys that they should walk over to the child to see what's wrong.

Attempt: They walk over to the crying child. Ashley asks whether they can help him. He says he does not know what happened to his father and their dog.

Plan: The group decides that three of them will go searching in the park for the dad and dog while Ashley stays with the boy.

Attempt: They break up and walk around various areas of the park searching for the dad and dog.

Consequence: Jim sees a man chasing a dog across the park; it looks like the dog's leash is broken.

Attempt: Jim runs to the man to ask if his son was with him. The man says yes, that he asked his son to stay by the park bench as he went after their dog. Jim says his friends found the boy crying. One of them is staying with him now.

Consequence: Jim and the man capture the dog and walk back to the boy and Ashley.

Reaction: The father is relieved to have his dog back on the leash. The boy is joyful that his father and dog have returned. Ashley calls Alexis on her cell phone to tell her that they found the boy's father and she and Tom can return to the boy. When the group has returned, the father thanks them for taking care of his son and helping him to stop his dog.

Codes: Sc, Rc, Ex, Pr, Ac, Hb, AL.

Glossary

Acquisition The initial learning of a skill.

Activity The range of experiences a person chooses or choices a person makes given a particular impairment.

Aid An object or device, either electronic or nonelectronic, used to transmit or receive messages; examples include communication books, eye-gaze frames, and computers.

Aided symbol A symbol that requires external support (e.g., an object or a picture displayed on a communication board or book or a picture or a word programmed into a device) and which cannot be expressed with or on the body.

American English (AE) The type of English spoken in the United States. As other languages, AE includes a number of different dialects.

Augmentative/alternative communication (AAC) Message transmission not achieved through conventional means (i.e., speech), but in any number of other ways, including, but not limited to, use of gestures, facial expressions, sign, communication boards, and various electronic or nonelectronic devices or aids.

Authentic assessment The modification of assessment procedures to make them more naturalistic or to reflect a realistic, natural context.

Autism spectrum disorder An impairment defined by a given set of limitations in communication; a restricted range of interests and deficits in social interaction.

Baseline The level of performance of a child before beginning treatment or the measurement of behavior in the absence of treatment.

Basic interpersonal communication skills (BICS) Language proficiency involved in context-embedded social interactions.

Benchmark The expectations for academic performance at a given grade level for a particular subject area.

Bilingualism The ability to speak two languages.

Bound morpheme A type of morpheme that has to be attached to a free morpheme to have meaning.

Child-centered approaches A type of treatment for child language disorders that are high in terms of naturalness and that follow a child's interest to facilitate communicative interaction.

Childhood aphasia A language impairment caused by a neurological insult.

Clinician-directed approaches A type of treatment for child language disorders that are low in terms of naturalness in which the clinician elicits a set of desired behaviors from the child in the context of discrete trials.

Code switching Also referred to as code mixing. A natural component of bilingualism, which refers to a speaker's use of a word, phrase, or sentence from one language or dialect when communicating in the other language or dialect.

Cognitive academic language proficiency (CALP) Language proficiency involved in context-reduced academic settings.

Cognitive impairment An impairment in the acquisition and development of concepts and language.

Cognitive referencing The use of intelligence quotient (IQ) as a comparison for other domains of development.

Communication The exchange of information. There is a sender, a receiver, and the information exchanged.

Communication board A low technology aid that displays symbols (e.g., words, pictures, photographs, and/or objects); an individual points to these symbols to convey messages.

Communicative intent A characteristic that is typically acquired during infancy demonstrated by behaviors such as vocalizing, gesturing, gaze coupling, and persisting that shows that the child actually means to communicate.

Comorbidity The occurrence or association of one or more behaviors or symptoms with a particular diagnosis.

Condition The set of circumstances under which a given behavior is expected.

Conjoining The linguistic process of adding a phrase or clause to a sentence in an equal role, which increases the complexity of the sentence.

Conjunction A word used to connect words, phrases, and clauses. Typically, a child begins conjoining using the conjunction *and*. As the typical child develops linguistically, other conjunctions are also used (e.g., *because, if, but, therefore*).

Continuum of naturalness An organizational contrivance for describing a wide range of eclectic treatment approaches for child language disorders based on their degree of naturalness.

Controlled investigation Treatment efficacy evidence growing out of controlled investigations is strong owing to the experimental control such that the gains associated with the treatment can be attributed to the treatment.

Conversational discourse A series of utterances from participants in a conversation.

Criterion Level of performance expected from a child for a given goal or objective.

Criterion referenced assessment A procedure that uses a set of predetermined skills to assess; the skills may be developmental or curriculum based.

Culturally and linguistically diverse (CLD) populations Individuals who differ from the Anglo-European mainstream Americans.

Culture Systems of knowledge, experiences, behaviors, beliefs, and values shared by a group of people.

Decontextualized language Language referring to people, events, and experiences not present in the immediate context.

Dependent variables The effects, or responses, presumed to be caused by the independent variables.

Derivational morpheme A morpheme used to construct new words; includes affixes that appear at the beginning or ends of words and change the word's meaning or part of speech by their presence (e.g., base word = *happy*; derivational morphemes *un-*, *-ness*; new word = *unhappy* and *happiness*).

Derivational suffixes A subset of derivational morphemes. Suffixes appear only at the ends of words and change word meaning or part of speech (e.g., *ly* added to *quick* results in *quickly*).

Developmental-social-pragmatic As described by Wetherby and Prizant, a set of treatment approaches that are child centered and that provide learning experiences in naturally occurring or naturalistic contexts.

Dialect Any variety of a language that is spoken by a group of individuals that reflects and is determined by shared social, cultural/ethnic, or regional factors.

Dialogic book reading An approach to promoting language development where the same book is read repeatedly so that it becomes familiar and the clinician progressively encourages participation on the child's part in a natural conversational style.

Direct replication studies Investigations whose findings are likely to generalize across subjects.

Direct selection Pointing directly to a symbol on an aid with a finger or other body part or with a head stick or light pointer attached to a person's body.

Discrete trials Structured opportunities for training. The term *discrete* is used because a pause is inserted between one opportunity and the next.

Disorder The posession of or having a condition that represents a departure from the typical or expected parameters for that condition.

Do-statement A description of specifically what a child will do to meet a goal or objective.

Down syndrome A genetic syndrome defined by the addition of more chromosomes in the chromosomal structure than are typical.

Dynamic assessment The modification of assessment procedures to determine the kinds of supports a child needs to succeed on a given item or task.

Educational benchmarks A set of skills and abilities expected of children in a particular academic area for a particular grade.

Eligibility When a child meets a certain set of criteria for a diagnostic label, then she is able to receive speech and language services.

Embedding The linguistic process of inserting a phrase or clause into a sentence in a subordinate role that makes that sentence more complex.

English-language learners (ELL) Students who come from language backgrounds other than English and whose English proficiency has not developed enough to fully follow the academic curriculum in English; hence, added instructional support is needed.

Enhanced milieu teaching The use of milieu teaching in conjunction with environmental arranging and responsive interacting.

Evidence-based practice An approach to clinical practice that integrates research evidence, clinical expertise, and patient values.

Exemplar A prototypical example that may serve as a reference point.

Expansion A form of recasting in which the clinician's restatement does not go beyond the child's initial meaning.

Expert opinion The lowest status on the hierarchy of treatment efficacy evidence. Therefore, when treatment has only this support, it should not be used.

Expository language The language found in many textbooks, which has concepts and information organized and presented in a particular structure.

Expressive language The polar opposite of receptive language. The language that has been encoded in preparation for conveying the message.

Extension A form of recasting in which the clinician's restatement does go beyond the initial meaning of the child's utterance to include additional semantic detail.

Extrinsic reinforcement A type of reinforcement that does not naturally occur during conversation such as giving tokens, stickers, and verbal praise.

Facilitative play A type of treatment for young children with language disorders where the clinician tries to entice the child into communicating but from the child's perspective it is just play.

Fading A technique used during treatment where prompts or models are gradually reduced as the child begins to acquire the target form.

Feedback A type of consequence where information regarding the correctness of the response is provided.

Figurative language Language whose meaning must be inferred by the listener and includes idioms, metaphors, similes, and proverbs.

Focused stimulation A technique for facilitating language development in children where the clinician provides repeated models of the target form in a meaningful communicative context.

Formulating language Also called encoding. The process of putting thoughts into linguistic form to express them.

Fragile X syndrome A genetic syndrome defined by differences in the X chromosomal structure.

General stimulation An approach to treating language disorders in young children where the clinician talks about what he or she is doing so the child sees a close correspondence between the clinician's words and actions.

Generalization The occurrence of behavior in contexts that have not been trained.

Genetic and chromosomal disorder A disorder caused by the inheritance of certain traits in the genetic makeup of an individual.

Goals A set of long-term and more general expectations developed for a child.

Grammatical morphemes As explained by Roger Brown, a particular set of morphemes believed to be significant for morphologic and syntactic development.

Hearing impairment A deficit in the reception of the auditory signal.

Hierarchy An organization of skills, abilities, stimuli, or stimulus contexts that starts with the easier component and progresses to increasingly more complex and difficult components.

High technology (high tech) Electronic/computerized augmentative/ alternative communication systems, which use synthesized speech and allow text-to-speech communication; aids accessible in multiple ways (e.g., pointing, switch use with scanning, infrared pointer).

Hybrid approach A type of treatment for child language disorders where the clinician borrows elements from both clinician-directed and client-centered approaches.

Hypothesis testing A form of logic used in the scientific method where an experiment is implemented to test the validity of a hypothesis.

Illocutionary An aspect of the spoken message that includes the intended effect by the speaker; infants may use nonsymbolic vocalizations with intent to request, protest, and so on.

Impairment The specific diagnostic category given to a particular person, for example, language disorder.

Incidental teaching A variation of milieu teaching where after a child initiates an interaction, the clinician requires elaboration before delivering the reinforcement.

Independent variables The presumed causative factors that operate on dependent variables.

Individualized education plan (IEP) The plan developed by an educational team to address the learning issues of a given child.

Intelligence quotient A measure of cognitive ability as determined by a child's performance on a particular set of standardized tests.

Interpreting language Also called decoding. The process of comprehending a linguistic message that has been received.

Intonation A prosodic feature, specifically the pitch envelope over the utterance length.

Intrinsic reinforcement A type of reinforcement that naturally arises in the communicative context, such as giving juice to a child who requests it.

Joint reference The child and caregiver focus simultaneously on the same event or object; also known as joint attention.

Language A system of symbols and rules for combining them to communicate a message.

Language-based learning disability An impairment in the acquisition and use of language, usually associated with typical cognitive abilities.

Language comprehension The understanding or recognition of a message presented by a speaker or read in text.

Language content *See* semantics.

Language delay The condition in which a child is developing language more slowly than expected.

Language deviance The presence of a language pattern that would be considered not typical for a child of any developmental level.

Language differences Individual's linguistic variations on one language that reflect regular patterns in the individual's primary language/dialect. Many cultural groups living in the United States will exhibit linguistic variations that reflect bilingual/bidialectal influences on English.

Language disorder The usual term used for a language impairment, a deficit in the comprehension or expression of language.

Language form The phonology, syntax, and morphology of language.

Language impairment The presence of a language abilities that are below expectations based on the child's age.

Language-learning disability (LLD) Disability that affects the individual's ability to learn any language. For an accurate diagnosis of LLD among bilingual individuals, language difficulties have to be evident in both languages.

Language loss Process observed among second-language learners where they tend to lose their first language if its use is decreased. Such language loss process has been observed as a shift in proficiency with second-language learners losing skills in the first language, as proficiency is acquired in the second language.

Language transference Common phenomenon observed among individuals who learn a second language in which they transfer the characteristics of their primary language into the second language. The various components of language can be transferred (i.e., syntax, phonology, morphology, semantics, and pragmatics).

Language use Pragmatics; how the child uses his knowledge of language in differing social contexts.

Linguistic parameters Dimensions of language identified by linguists and include phonology, semantics, syntax, morphology, and pragmatics.

Locutionary An aspect of the spoken message that includes the underlying meaning as reflected in the syntax and semantic elements of the sentence.

Low technology (low tech) Augmentative/alternative communication devices that do not use electricity or electronics but may use a battery and store recorded messages; also includes simple communication aids, such as boards or books with various types of symbols (e.g., letters, pictures, phrases, and words).

Maintenance The review of previously acquired skills so that they are not lost.

Mand-model An extension of incidental teaching where the clinician requests a verbal response from the child. If it is not forthcoming, the clinician models the target behavior and asks the child to repeat it.

Mapping Labeling or symbolizing each concept with a word.

Mean The average of a set of scores.

Mean length of utterance The average length of an utterance in a language sample determined by counting the number of morphemes in each utterance.

Mean length of utterance-2 As described by Johnston, this method removes utterances from the sample that are imitative, utterances that are single-word *yes/no* responses, and any utterances that are elliptical responses to a question.

Mediate generalization A method of facilitating generalization of a training target by teaching the child the rule for applying a certain behavior. Then the clinician relies on the child's self-management skills to do so. For example, assume that the training target is greeting behavior. The child is taught the rule "When you see a friend for the first time in the day, greet that person."

Metalinguistic ability The ability to consciously reflect on language.

Metaphor A type of figurative language in which one referent is described in terms of another.

Milieu teaching A general approach to facilitating language acquisition in which operant conditioning principles are applied in a quasi-natural setting.

Model A correct production of the target response for the child to imitate.

Morpheme The smallest linguistic unit in speech that has meaning.

Morphology A linguistic parameter concerned with word forms and inflections.

Narrative discourse A form of speech that differs from conversational discourse in that it is typically a monologue requiring greater structure and coherence.

Narratives A type of text that describes an event or tells a story.

Nonword repetition The repetition of nonsense words, believed to be a nonbiased means of assessing language processing.

Normative sample The sample of children who take a test to determine how typical children perform on a given standardized test.

No-tech systems Augmentative/alternative communication systems, including gestures, sign language, or eye gaze alone.

Number of different words The number of different words observed in a language sample.

Number of total words The number of total words used by a child in a language sample.

Objective Short-term, very specific expectations for a given child's performance.

Overextension Use of a word to encompass a broader meaning than permitted in adult language (e.g., *Kitty* referring to all cats, lions, and tigers).

Participation How societal and cultural norms and laws are established to support the participation of a person with an impairment.

Peer reviewed A designation that an article has passed a rigorous review process that reduces the potential for misinformation.

Perlocutionary An aspect of the spoken message that includes the effect of an utterance on its recipient; for infants who communicate unintentionally, meaning is ascribed to their vocalizations by caregivers.

Personal narrative A form of discourse for telling others a story about oneself.

Phonemes The individual speech sounds, including both the vowels and consonants, that differentiate spoken words.

Phonemic awareness The knowledge of the way phonemes and morphemes are combined to make syllables and words and to convey meaning.

Phonology A linguistic parameter referring to the speech sounds.

Prader-Willi syndrome A genetic syndrome defined by differences in the chromosomal structure of the 15th chromosome.

Pragmatics A linguistic parameter addressing the rules governing the use of language in social context.

Prelinguistic milieu teaching A variation of milieu teaching in which clear, frequent, nonverbal communication, such as vocalizing, gazing, and pointing, is promoted.

Prevalence The number of people who have a particular condition or diagnosis at a particular time.

Prognosis The predicted outcome of a course of treatment.

Program common stimuli A method of facilitating generalization of a training target by bringing salient elements from the natural communicative environment into the training sessions. Bringing the child's peers into the training sessions would be an example.

Prompts Requests, hints, or cues designed to elicit the target response.

Prosodic features The speech sounds, unlike the phonemes, which vary over the length of the utterance and include stress, intonation, and rhythm.

Recasting A technique for facilitating language acquisition in which the clinician corrects a child's utterance by restating it in a fashion that only the corrective portion of the restatement is novel. As such, a minimal burden is placed on the child's memory.

Receptive language The polar opposite of expressive language. The language interpreted by the receiver of the message.

Reinforcement A type of consequence that increases the frequency of the behavior.

Reliability The degree to which a given score by a particular child will be obtained again with readmission of the same test.

Response to intervention (RtI) approach A multistep approach, which evaluates a child's ability to learn when provided with appropriate instruction. The child's progress is closely monitored and used for educational decisions. It is considered a prevention model mandated in the Individuals with Disabilities Education Improvement Act of 2004 as a way to minimize the overrepresentation of certain groups of students in special education.

Rett syndrome A neurodevelopmental disorder found almost exclusively in girls; one of the diagnoses on the autism spectrum.

Rhythm A prosodic feature involving stress timing that imparts a beat to spoken language.

Scaled score A score used to determine how a child's performance is distributed relative to the normative sample.

Scanning An indirect technique used to access a computer or communication aid that requires an individual to activate a switch for selection of the desired output, presented to the individual automatically; in partner-assisted scanning, the communication partner manually scans the choices for the AAC user and confirms with him or her the desired selection.

Script training An approach to promoting social interaction and associated language where thematic play using reciprocal roles such as doctor–patient, waitress–customer, and so on, serves as a context for rehearsal.

Semantics A linguistic parameter referring to the meaning dimension of language.

Sequential modification A method of facilitating generalization of a training target where the clinician checks in each environment to see if the target occurs. If it does not, then the target is trained in that environment.

Shaping A technique for training more complex responses, which involves gradually modifying a response in stages until eventually the target response is elicited.

Silent period A period that some second-language learners go through, characterized by little verbal output. During this period, second-language learners seem to be concentrating on listening, comprehending, learning the rules of the second language, and, many times, covertly rehearsing what they are learning.

Single subject design A methodology that focuses on individual variability under experimental conditions as a means of attributing the change in the target behavior to the treatment.

Sociodramatic play Children 3 to 5 years old engage in this pretend play using reciprocal roles embedded in themes (e.g., parent-child, doctor-patient and so on).

Specific language impairment (SLI) A language impairment that appears in individuals with typical cognitive abilities.

Speech The use of the vocal tract to express the encoded message.

Speech generating device A computerized or electronic device that provides speech output for individuals; this is often synthesized speech that allows for text to speech; also referred to as a voice output communication aid (*see* VOCA).

Standard deviation Determines how a score varies from the mean score of the normative sample.

Standard error of measure The degree to which a measurement obtained from a test varies from the true performance of the child.

Stimulus condition The context in which a given stimulus will be used; the kind of stimulus that will be used to elicit a particular response.

Strategy A method of using AAC (its symbols, aids, and techniques) to effectively convey a message; this may be accomplished by enhancing the timing, rate, or content of the message.

Stress A prosodic feature where extra strength or loudness is placed on some linguistic unit such as a syllable or word.

Symbol Something that stands for something else, its referent. There is an arbitrary relationship between the symbol and the referent. They are linked by community consensus.

Syntax A linguistic parameter referring to the rules of word order for phrases, clauses, and sentences.

Systematically replicated studies Investigations whose findings are likely to generalize across different investigators, settings, and subjects.

Target response The behavior or form that is being taught.

Techniques Methods for transmitting symbols for communication; these include but are not limited to gesturing, signing, pointing with a finger or head stick, various types of scanning (e.g., directed, linear, row-column), and encoding.

Therapeutic register A variation in speech used by speech-language pathologists to accommodate to a child's age and diagnostic status.

Time delay An extension of incidental teaching where the clinician uses a strategic pause to prompt the child to initiate an utterance.

Training stimuli The materials such as pictures or objects that are used for eliciting responses during training.

Traumatic brain injury An acquired neurobehavioral condition that results from an insult or injury to the brain.

Treatment efficacy The power of a treatment to change behavior.

Tuberous sclerosis A genetic disease that results in the growth of benign tumors in the brain and other vital organs.

T-unit A terminal unit, a main clause, and all of the associated subordinate clauses and phrases.

Type/token ratio A measure of vocabulary diversity, determined by comparing the total number of words to the number of different words in a language sample.

Unaided symbol A symbol expressed or on the body, such as speech, gestures, and sign, requiring no external support.

Uncontrolled investigation Treatment efficacy evidence that is weak owing to the lack of experimental control. Therefore, gains associated with the treatment cannot actually be attributed to the treatment.

Underextension Use of a word to encompass a narrower meaning than seen in adult language (e.g., *doggie* used only for the child's pet but not for other dogs).

Utterance A group of words expressed by a child to communicate meaning; may be a single word, a phrase or a sentence.

Validity The degree to which a test actually assesses the abilities it claims to assess.

Vertical restructuring A type of expansion occurring over multiple conversational turns and provides a model of the multiword target utterance.

Violating object's function A means of increasing a child's need to communicate by using an object with an obvious function in an inappropriate fashion. For example, an adult is preparing a bowl of Cheerios but has placed the bowl upside down.

Violating routine events A means of increasing a child's need to communicate by first establishing a routine with expectations; for example, rolling a ball back and forth. Then, the adult fails to roll the ball back as expected.

Vocal tract The speech structures (e.g., the larynx, tongue, and lips) used to create speech.

Voice output communication aid (VOCA) A computerized or electronic device that provides voice output for individuals; also referred to as a speech generating device; some may be dedicated (i.e., used solely for communication) and others, such as computers, may fulfill multiple functions.

Withholding objects A means of increasing a child's need to communicate by withholding an object that is needed for an activity. For example, the child is ready to start coloring. Everything is available except for the crayons. The crayons are in the child's line of sight but out of reach.

Zone of proximal development The learning edge of a child; the area where skills or abilities are just beginning to develop, but are not mastered, and can be observed by structuring assessment procedures to support the performance of a child.

INDEX

Note: Tables are noted with a *t*.